PRESS HERE!

FACE WORKOUTS
~FOR BEGINNERS~

PRESS HERE!

FACE WORKOUTS

~FOR BEGINNERS~

PRESSURE TECHNIQUES TO TONE AND DEFINE NATURALLY

NADIRA V PERSAUD

FAIR WINDS

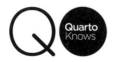

Inspiring | Educating | Creating | Entertaining

Brimming with creative inspiration, how-to projects, and useful information to enrich your everyday life, Quarto Knows is a favorite destination for those pursuing their interests and passions. Visit our site and dig deeper with our books into your area of interest: Quarto Creates, Quarto Cooks, Quarto Homes, Quarto Lives, Quarto Drives, Quarto Explores, Quarto Gifts, or Quarto Kids.

First Published in 2020 by Fair Winds Press, an imprint of The Quarto Group. 100 Cummings Center, Suite 265-D, Beverly, MA 01915, USA. T (978) 282-9590 F (978) 283-2742

Fair Winds Press titles are also available at discount for retail, wholesale, promotional, and bulk purchase. For details, contact the Special Sales Manager by email at specialsales@quarto.com or by mail at The Quarto Group, Attn: Special Sales Manager, 100 Cummings Center, Suite 265-D, Beverly, MA 01915, USA.

23 22 21 20 24 1 2 3 4 5

ISBN: 978-1-59233-942-6

Digital edition published in 2020

QUAR.327858

Conceived, edited, and designed by
Quarto Publishing plc. 6 Blundell Street,
London N7 9BH

Editor: Claire Waite Brown
Senior art editor: Emma Clayton
Designer: Joanna Bettles
Illustrator: Kuo Kang Chen
Publisher: Samantha Warrington

Printed in Singapore.

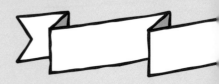

CONTENTS

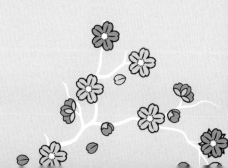

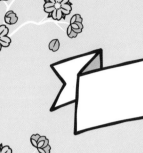

WELCOME

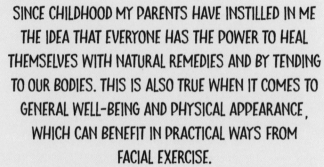

SINCE CHILDHOOD MY PARENTS HAVE INSTILLED IN ME THE IDEA THAT EVERYONE HAS THE POWER TO HEAL THEMSELVES WITH NATURAL REMEDIES AND BY TENDING TO OUR BODIES. THIS IS ALSO TRUE WHEN IT COMES TO GENERAL WELL-BEING AND PHYSICAL APPEARANCE, WHICH CAN BENEFIT IN PRACTICAL WAYS FROM FACIAL EXERCISE.

This self-help process is now a big part of my personal and professional life, and I am wholeheartedly of the opinion that quick fixes aren't the solution. Instead, I know that regular and consistent beauty routines embedded into everyday life can pave the way to optimum results, namely toned, defined, and well-rested skin.

After more than twenty years as a makeup artist it is this holistic approach to beauty that I continue to offer to my clients, from everyday women and men to celebrities. While I have built my portfolio of work in television, advertising, fashion, and beauty, I also share my knowledge with international beauty companies as a brand consultant, as well as contributing to top glossy and industry editorials in print and online.

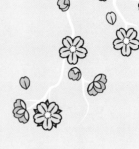

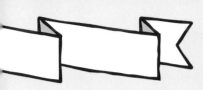

My outlook is about enhancing natural beauty at the same time as concentrating on lifestyle, to strike a balance between looking and feeling good. Alongside this philosophy I continue to celebrate each and every face I work with by actively sharing step-by-step routines. I am now very happy to be able to share these exercises with you, and hope that you will benefit in multiple ways from my effective and efficient skincare advice based on practice and routine.

This book features a collection of workouts comprised of a number of facial exercises that will glean the best results if they are carried out regularly and in the order detailed. Within each workout different techniques are used—such as massage and sweeping the skin to pressing and holding on various points of the face—in order to release tension, promote blood flow, and disperse fluid: crucial elements for toning and improving face structure and quality.

66 *It's beauty that captures your attention; personality which captures your heart.* 99

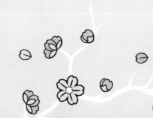

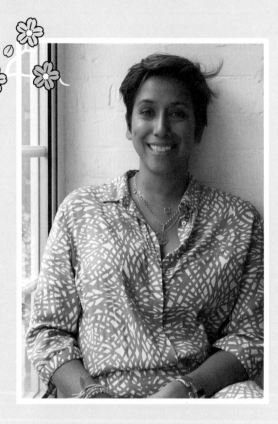

The workouts themselves can be performed in any order, although given the nature of the workout called Warm Up and Wake Up (see pages 22–35), this one is best performed first thing in the morning as an awakening routine.

While it is recommended that you complete the exercises within a workout in the order given, you are not expected to complete all of the workouts in a single session (although you are welcome to if you wish). If you want to target a specific area, simply choose the workout that correlates. Remember that problem areas will benefit best from being exercised regularly, with daily being the ideal scenario.

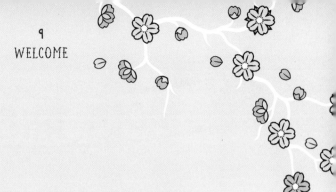

I have also put together two express workouts (see pages 122–125), for those time-poor yet crucial moments when you want to pep-up glow or de-stress. These workouts are standalone, but equally can be performed along with the other workouts.

Once you become familiar with the workouts you will no doubt hit upon your favorite combination, and find you can fit them into your everyday routine more easily and consistently. You will soon see the benefits of your new exercise regime.

Nadira V Persaud

DISCLAIMER

It is the sole responsibility of the individual to decide whether these exercises are suitable for them. If you have any medical issues past, present, or ongoing please consult your doctor or physician, especially if you are in a post-recovery period.

Extreme pressure must not be applied to the temples or in and around the eye area.

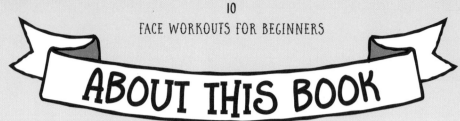

ABOUT THIS BOOK

This book guides the reader through a simple step-by-step process for each exercise within each workout. Invest time in these workouts and you will reap the rewards.

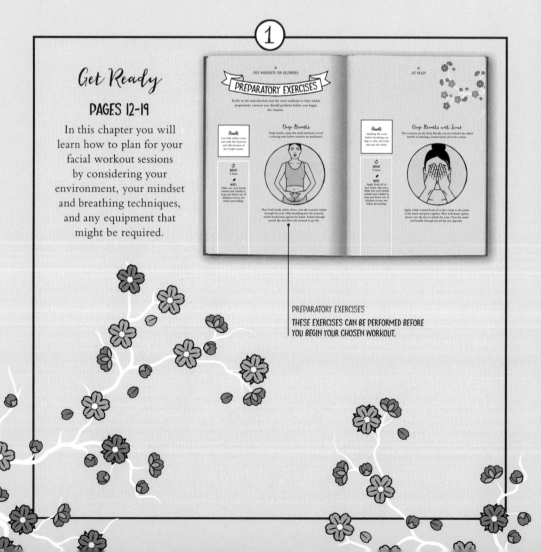

Get Ready

PAGES 12-19

In this chapter you will learn how to plan for your facial workout sessions by considering your environment, your mindset and breathing techniques, and any equipment that might be required.

PREPARATORY EXERCISES
THESE EXERCISES CAN BE PERFORMED BEFORE YOU BEGIN YOUR CHOSEN WORKOUT.

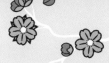

The Workouts

PAGES 20–119

These workouts are designed to target particular areas of the face—such as the eyes, mouth area, and skin. Follow the flow of exercises, which are best performed in the order given.

THE INFORMATION GIVEN IN THESE PANELS IS INTENDED TO PROVIDE THE BEST-CASE SCENARIO. IT IS IMPORTANT TO WORK WITHIN YOUR MEANS AND WITH WHAT YOU HAVE. SO, IF YOU HAVE LESS TIME AVAILABLE, YOU CAN STILL DO THE EXERCISE, BUT CUT IT SHORT. IF YOU DON'T HAVE A MIRROR OR FACE CREAM THESE EXERCISES ARE STILL FOR YOU. MODIFY WHERE YOU MUST AND ENJOY!

INTRODUCTION
THE INTRODUCTION TO EACH EXERCISE PROVIDES VITAL INSIGHT INTO WHAT HAPPENS DURING THE PROCESS.

STEPS
ILLUSTRATIONS AND DETAILED TEXT MAKE THE EXERCISE EASY TO REPLICATE.

BENEFITS
SEE AT A GLANCE THE BENEFITS EACH EXERCISE IMPARTS.

Express Workouts

PAGES 120–125

The two express workouts have been put together using a number of the exercises from the previous chapters, combined in a unique order to target two common concerns.

ROUTINE
FOLLOW THESE EXERCISES IN THE ORDER PROVIDED.

STEPS
A CONDENSED DESCRIPTION OF THE EXERCISE IS GIVEN, WITH A CROSS-REFERENCE TO THE FULL EXERCISE.

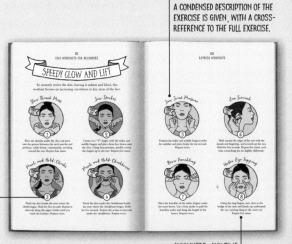

ANYWHERE, ANY TIME
THESE EXERCISES HAVE BEEN MODIFIED, AND CAN BE PERFORMED WITHOUT EQUIPMENT.

GET READY

THE FOLLOWING PAGES PROVIDE GUIDELINES TO HELP YOU PREPARE FOR THE WORKOUTS, WHICH SHOULD BE PERFORMED IN THE BEST ENVIRONMENT FOR YOU, WHETHER SEATED OR STANDING, WITH ALL CHOSEN EQUIPMENT CLOSE BY. READ THROUGH EACH EXERCISE BEFORE ENGAGING TO FULLY UNDERSTAND THE MOTION AND TECHNIQUE. YOU WILL FIND THAT, OVER TIME, THE ROUTINES BECOME SECOND NATURE.

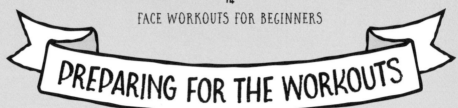

PREPARING FOR THE WORKOUTS

These exercises can be performed almost anywhere, although you will get the most out of the workouts if you perform them in an uninterrupted space. For each exercise I have set out to guide you toward the ideal environment to get the best out of the techniques.

Standing or Seated

Most of the exercises can be performed either standing or seated. Occasionally, an exercise may be better performed seated, for example to allow your elbows to rest on a surface for support.

In Front of a Mirror

You will benefit from using a mirror when stated to ensure positioning is accurate; however, over time and through regular practice, you might find the mirror unnecessary.

With Eyes Closed

Keeping the eyes closed during some exercises is suggested so that you can concentrate on your breath and on releasing tension. Though this is not a rule that has to be applied, it is recommended. Once new confidence is found through practice you may find you naturally close your eyes during some exercises.

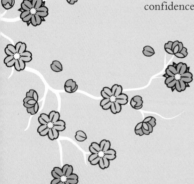

Out and About

Exercises that don't require hand contact with the face can be executed anywhere, for example waiting at the bus stop or during a lunch break.

Props and Equipment

Facial oils and face creams, as well as eye products, are listed as ideal equipment for some exercises. Using them will mean you get the maximum effect from techniques such as gliding or knuckling, since a little slip can avoid dragging or pulling the skin. However, it is entirely your choice whether to use skin products or not.

You might choose to perform a workout as part of your skincare routine, as a way of applying your daily moisturizer or eye cream.

Breathing and Inhibitions

In the workouts chapters a recommendation to breathe through certain exercises is sometimes given, to ensure the face and body maintain a relaxed disposition. This is usually most relevant during knuckling and press-and-hold techniques. Practicing breathing deeply and slowly is highly advised (see page 16).

You should also make every effort to let go of self-conscious feelings. This ideal mindset will help you to fully engage when articulating an exercise, and rid your face and body of tension.

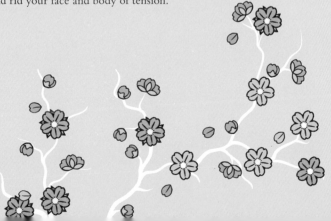

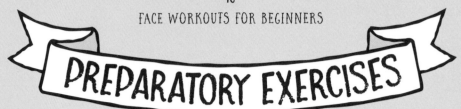

PREPARATORY EXERCISES

Refer to the introduction text for each workout to find which preparatory exercise you should perform before you begin the routine.

Benefits

Can help reduce stress and assist the function and effectiveness of the lymph system.

REPEAT
5 times

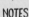

NOTES
Make sure each breath inhaled and exhaled is long and drawn out. If dizziness occurs, rest before proceeding.

Deep Breaths

Deep breaths center the mind and body toward a relaxing state before exercises are performed.

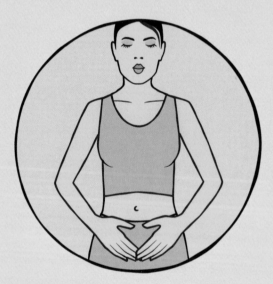

Place both hands, palms down, over the stomach. Inhale through the nose while breathing into the stomach, which should push against the hands. Exhale through pursed lips and allow the stomach to go flat.

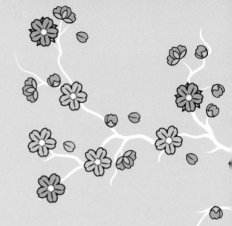

Benefits

Inhaling the scent before breathing can help to relax the body and ease the mind.

REPEAT
5 times

NOTES
Apply facial oil or face cream only once. Make sure each breath inhaled and exhaled is long and drawn out. If dizziness occurs, rest before proceeding.

Deep Breaths with Scent

This variation on the Deep Breaths exercise includes the added benefit of inhaling a scented facial oil or face cream.

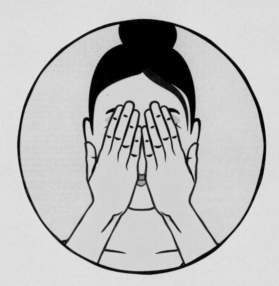

Apply a little scented facial oil or face cream to the palms of the hands and press together. Place both hands (palms down) over the face to inhale the scent. Clear the mind and breathe through pursed lips (see opposite).

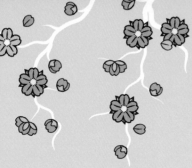

Shoulder Rolls

Stress can be felt in the shoulders, so loosening the muscles in this area helps you to feel grounded and improves posture.

Benefits

Releases tension and acknowledges alignment in the body.

REPEAT

3 times forward,
3 times back

NOTES

Do not perform if you have nerve pain in the neck or shoulder areas.

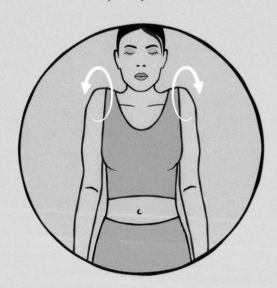

With your arms by your sides, slowly circle the shoulders so they travel up to the ears and round to the back. Repeat three times.

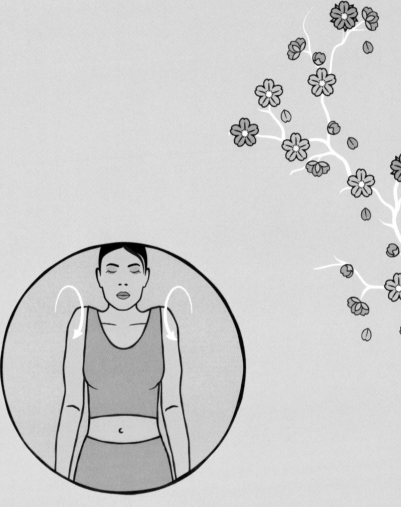

Now roll the shoulders in the opposite direction,
traveling up to the ears, then forward. Repeat
three times.

WARM UP AND WAKE UP

THIS INITIAL SEQUENCE OF WARM-UP EXERCISES FOR THE ENTIRE FACE WAKES UP MUSCLES AND IMPROVES CIRCULATION, MAKING IT AN IDEAL DAILY MORNING ROUTINE.

———————————————

BEGIN THIS WORKOUT WITH DEEP BREATHS AND SHOULDER ROLLS (SEE PAGES 16 AND 18-19).

NECK STRETCH

The neck can be a delicate area and subject to tension if you are under stress or have sleep issues, which is why this gentle stretch is a vital part of your daily routine.

Benefits
Releases tension in the neck and helps to loosen any stiffness.

REPEAT
Once on each side

TIME
30 seconds

ENVIRONMENT
Standing or seated. In front of a mirror

EQUIPMENT
None

NOTES
Keep shoulders down so as not to create strain. Only go as far as feels comfortable, and don't forget to breathe.

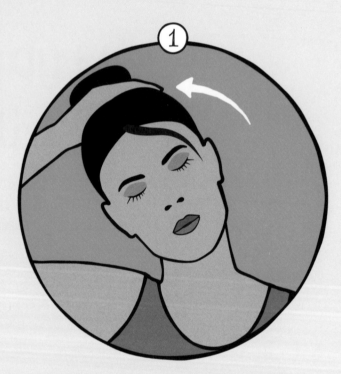

Standing tall, place the left hand over the head, positioning it above the right ear. Gently move the head toward the left shoulder for the stretch on the right side of the neck. Hold for 10–15 seconds.

Repeat the exercise with the right hand to stretch the left side of the neck.

FULL-FACE MOTION

Stress and tensions in the face can lead to puffiness and manifest in lack of tone in the complexion. Being facially engaged keeps muscles activated and stimulated.

Benefits

Quickly relaxes the facial muscles and releases tension in the jaw.

REPEAT
5 times

TIME
Up to 10 seconds

ENVIRONMENT
Standing or seated. In front of a mirror

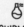

EQUIPMENT
None

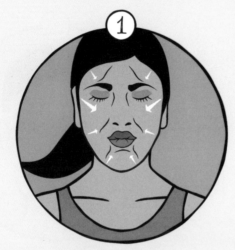

Screw up the face and eyes as tightly as possible.

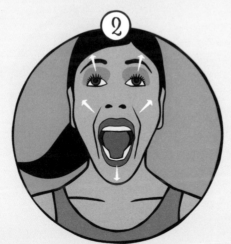

Quickly release, allowing the eyes and mouth to open as wide as possible.

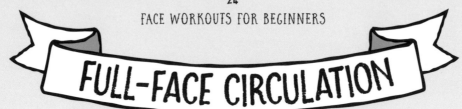

FULL-FACE CIRCULATION

Tension is commonly held around the mouth during times of stress and crisis, which can lead to "trauma lines" beside the mouth and deterioration of elasticity. By reenergizing the area around the mouth, deep lines can be avoided.

Benefits
Releases tension around the mouth, leaving a softer contour that, over time, helps to avoid deep lines.

REPEAT
5 times clockwise, 5 times counterclockwise

TIME
20 seconds

ENVIRONMENT
Standing or seated. In front of a mirror

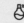

EQUIPMENT
None

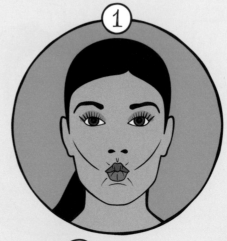

Purse the lips tightly together.

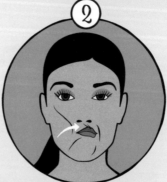

Slowly move the mouth in a circular motion, concentrating on keeping the motion fully articulated. Make five circles in a clockwise direction.

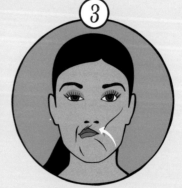

Make five circles counterclockwise.

FACE ACTIVATOR

Some facial muscles are less engaged than others, but this exercise offers full-face activation. It also wakes up the throat, so is ideal for those with thyroid issues.

Benefits
Fully wakes up the face and throat.

REPEAT
5 times

TIME
20 seconds

ENVIRONMENT
Standing or seated.
In front of a mirror

EQUIPMENT
None

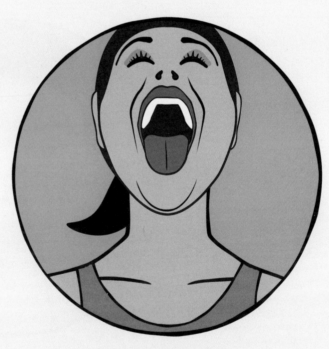

Open the eyes and mouth wide, stick out the tongue, and make the sound "ahhh" from the back of the throat.

EYE SWEEPS

Lack of sleep and imbalances in specific organs can cause fluid retention around the eyes, leading to puffiness. Due to the delicate nature of the skin, this is often where we notice the first signs of aging.

Benefits

This is a lymphatic drainage exercise that offers a reduction in fluid retention with instant results.

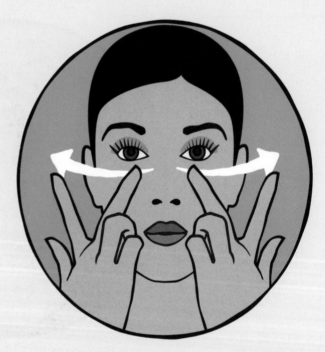

REPEAT
10 times

TIME
10 seconds

ENVIRONMENT
Standing or seated. In front of a mirror

EQUIPMENT
Eye cream or serum

NOTES
Ensure pressure is gentle, as if quickly sweeping the surface of the skin.

Apply eye cream or serum to the area under the eyes. Place the middle fingers under each eye close to the nose, then gently sweep outward.

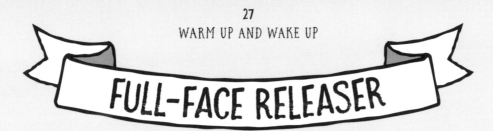

FULL-FACE RELEASER

Breathing techniques help to ease tension and improve circulation, while expanding the cheeks is an efficient workout.

Benefits
Tones the face from the inside out.

REPEAT
5 times

TIME
30 seconds

ENVIRONMENT
Standing or seated.
In front of a mirror

EQUIPMENT
None

NOTES
Ensure cheeks and area around the mouth are fully expanded with air.

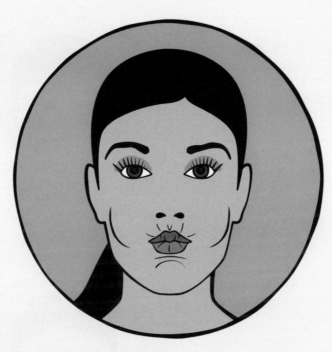

With shoulders back and relaxed, breathe in and hold the breath with the cheeks filled and puffed out. Hold for approximately five seconds.

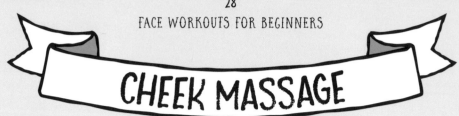

FACE WORKOUTS FOR BEGINNERS

CHEEK MASSAGE

A lot of tension is held in the cheeks—especially the hard-to-reach areas such as under the cheekbones—which can lead to deep lines or reduced tone and bone structure.

Benefits

This exercise offers instant relief under the cheekbones, and immediate toning.

REPEAT
Twice

TIME
20 seconds

ENVIRONMENT
Standing or seated.
In front of a mirror

EQUIPMENT
None

NOTES
Ensure reasonable pressure is applied for optimum results.

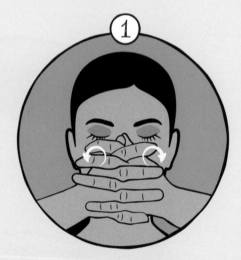

Gently interlock the fingers and place the hands over the face with the thenar (the fleshy part of the hand at the base of the thumb) pressed under the cheekbones close to the nose. Use small circular movements of the thenar to slowly massage all along the cheekbones.

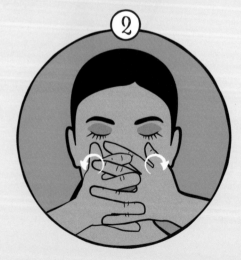

As you work farther away from the nose you can unlock the fingers to continue the massage.

FOREHEAD MASSAGE

Simple massage techniques can relieve headaches or unwanted tension behind the eyes. They can also ease tightness on the forehead, which leads to frown lines and deep horizontal lines.

Benefits
Instant relief and good for avoiding lines if practiced regularly.

REPEAT
Twice

TIME
10 seconds

ENVIRONMENT
Standing or seated

EQUIPMENT
None

NOTES
If performing to relieve headaches, work slowly and repeat until some tension is released.

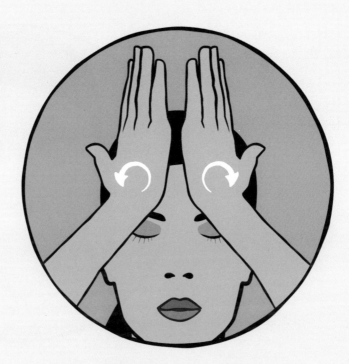

Place the hands on the forehead. Confidently press the thenar (the fleshy part of the hand at the base of the thumb) into the skin using circular motions, working from the center out.

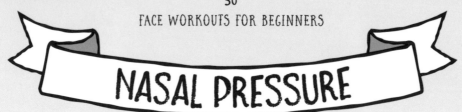

NASAL PRESSURE

Simply pressing down onto pressure points can achieve instant relief,
while applying firm pressure to tender spots helps to oxygenate
the area and disperse fluid.

Benefits

Tension is instantly
relieved. Can help
to de-puff the area
under the eyes.

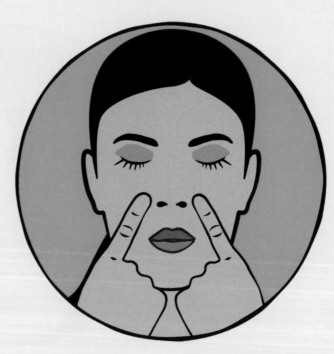

REPEAT
Press and hold for
10 seconds, or until
there is relief

TIME
10 seconds

ENVIRONMENT
Standing or seated

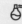

EQUIPMENT
None

NOTES
Take deep breaths
throughout this
exercise.

Place the index fingers over the tender points beside the
nasal passage. Press down firmly and hold.

INNER EYE PRESSURE

Applying pressure to specific pressure points helps banish tension, relieve stress, and force balance.

Benefits

Helps to de-puff around the eyes and improve eye contours. Offers instant relief for tension headaches and eye strain.

REPEAT

Press and hold for 10 seconds, or until there is relief

TIME

10 seconds

ENVIRONMENT

Standing or seated

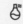

EQUIPMENT

None

NOTES

Take deep, steady breaths throughout this exercise. Hands can be unclasped also.

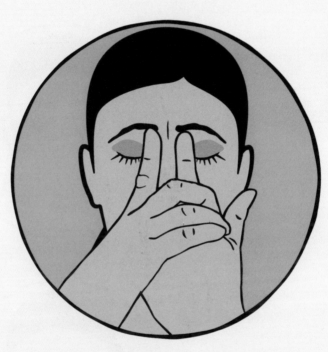

Place the index fingers just under each inner brow bone with clasped hands for even pressure. Find the tender spot, then press firmly and hold.

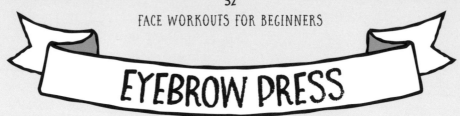

EYEBROW PRESS

It is common to feel tension around the eyes and forehead. Applying pressure along the brows can help relieve tension and promote a brighter, wide-eyed expression.

Benefits

Instant relief for tension headaches. Activates underused muscles.

REPEAT

Press and hold for 5 seconds at each point along the brow

TIME

20 seconds

ENVIRONMENT

Standing or seated

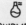

EQUIPMENT

None

NOTES

Don't forget to breathe deeply and steadily through the tension.

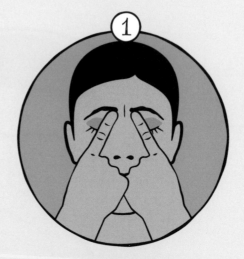

Place the index fingers onto each inner brow. Press firmly and hold for five seconds.

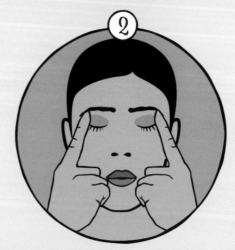

Repeat, moving the fingers along the brow a little each time. The final press should be made just before the temples.

FOREHEAD PRESS

Foreheads can show the visible signs of trauma and stress that our bodies feel, as well as revealing deep expression lines. This exercise assists consciousness of how not to engage in negative expressions, such as frowning.

Benefits

Relieves tension in the forehead and energizes the area. Activates underused muscles.

REPEAT
Press and hold for 5 seconds at each point along the forehead

TIME
20 seconds

ENVIRONMENT
Standing or seated

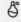

EQUIPMENT
None

NOTES
Breathe through any tension. Do not press directly onto the temples. The exercise can be repeated to ease tension headaches.

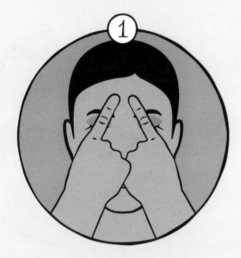

Place the index fingers at the center of the forehead. Press firmly and hold for five seconds.

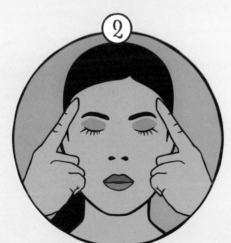

Repeat, moving the fingers along the forehead a little each time. The final press should be made just before the temples.

HAIR PULLING

Stimulating the scalp in this way activates blood flow to wake up the mind, body, and spirit.

Benefits
Instantly wakes up the scalp.

REPEAT
Tug for 1 second at each point around the scalp

TIME
Up to 15 seconds

ENVIRONMENT
Standing or seated

EQUIPMENT
None

NOTES
If there is no hair to pull, or you have current hair-loss issues, use the tips of the fingers to tap firmly over the scalp.

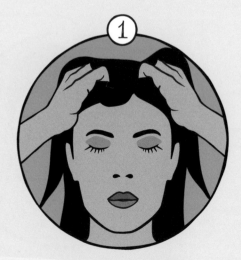

Grab a handful of hair firmly and tug for one second.

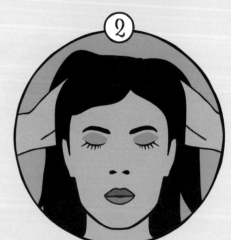

Repeat the same process over the entire head.

HEAD MASSAGE

Deep stimulation of the scalp activates blood flow, leading to that wide-awake feeling.

Benefits

Relieves tensions and can promote hair growth.

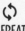
REPEAT
Repeat massage over entire head

TIME
Up to 1 minute

ENVIRONMENT
Standing or seated

EQUIPMENT
None

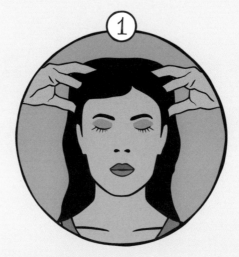

Press the tips of the fingers firmly into the scalp and make tiny circular motions.

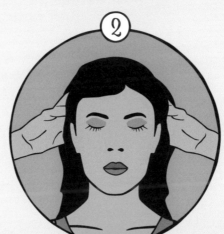

Keep contact with the skin while moving around the head.

FUNDAMENTAL FACE WORKOUT

MANIPULATION AND PRESSURE TECHNIQUES USED IN THIS WORKOUT PROVIDE IMMEDIATE RELEASE OF MUSCULAR TENSIONS. A FOCUS ON BREATHING IS IMPORTANT, WHICH CAN BE HELPED BY CLOSING THE EYES. THE NECK AND CHEST MOTIONS HELP TO INCREASE CIRCULATION TO REENERGIZE AND AID DISPERSION OF TOXINS, WHILE THE ATTENTION TO THE JAWLINE AND EARS ADDS MUCH RELIEF TO STIFF, MINISCULE MUSCLES AND JOINTS, WHICH LEADS TO IMPROVEMENTS IN SKIN QUALITY, TEXTURE, AND TONE.

START THIS WORKOUT WITH DEEP BREATHS AND SHOULDER ROLLS (SEE PAGES 16 AND 18-19).

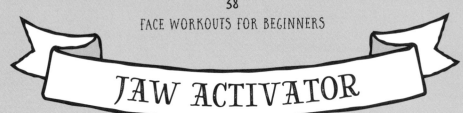

JAW ACTIVATOR

Initial pressure on the jaw can be surprisingly tender, so start with this short wake-up exercise.

Benefits

Reduction of fluid and tension. Improved quality of skin and definition to the jawline.

REPEAT
Twice

TIME
Up to 2 minutes

ENVIRONMENT
Standing or seated. In front of a mirror. With eyes closed

EQUIPMENT
Facial oil or face cream

NOTES
Do not perform if the area is swollen or tender to touch, or after dental care.

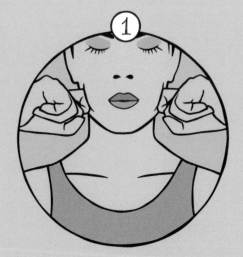

Smooth facial oil or cream over the face and neck. Bend the index fingers, then press the knuckles confidently onto the jawline, under the earlobes. Hold for up to three seconds. Release.

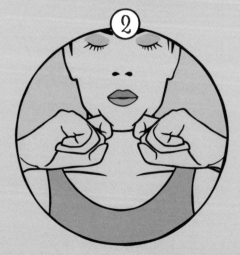

Move the knuckles along the jawline a little and repeat the hold. Continue all along the jaw.

OPEN JAW ACTIVATOR

A similar exercise to the Jaw Activator (opposite), this one features increased articulation to offer more toning to the jawline.

Benefits

Reduction of fluid and tension. Improved quality of skin and definition to the jawline.

REPEAT
Twice

TIME
Up to 2 minutes

ENVIRONMENT
Standing or seated. In front of a mirror. With eyes closed

EQUIPMENT
Facial oil or face cream

NOTES
Do not perform if the area is swollen or tender to touch, or after dental care.

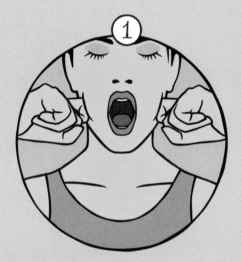

Smooth facial oil or cream over the face and neck. Bend the index fingers, then press the knuckles confidently onto the jawline, under the earlobes. As you press, open your mouth. Hold for up to three seconds. Release.

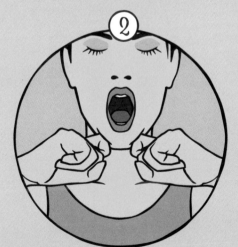

Move the knuckles along the jawline a little and repeat the hold. Continue all along the jaw.

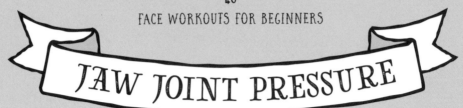

JAW JOINT PRESSURE

This press-and-hold exercise effectively releases tightness around the jaw, and precisely attends to common jaw conditions such as lockjaw and teeth grinding.

Benefits

Relieves constricted muscles at the joint to allow the jaw to move more freely.

REPEAT
Twice

TIME
20 seconds

ENVIRONMENT
Standing or seated. In front of a mirror. With eyes closed

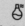

EQUIPMENT
None

NOTES
Do not perform if pain is immediate when pressed, or after dental care.

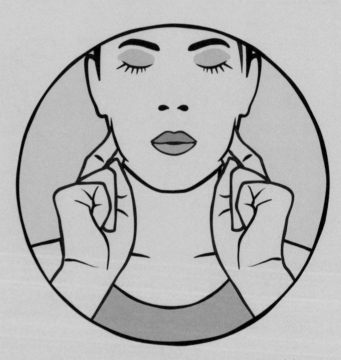

Position the index and middle fingers under the earlobes and press firmly for ten seconds.

JAWLINE PINCH

Pinching the skin on the jawline stimulates circulation. The gripping of the skin also assists in finding nodules of tension.

Benefits
Releases stiffness and activates blood flow through the skin.

REPEAT
Twice

TIME
Up to 1 minute

ENVIRONMENT
Standing or seated. In front of a mirror. With eyes closed

EQUIPMENT
None

NOTES
Do not perform if the area is swollen or tender to touch, or after dental care.

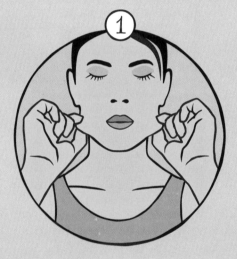

Starting under the earlobes, firmly pinch the skin on the jaw between the index fingers and thumbs, feeling a tug on the muscle. Hold for five seconds.

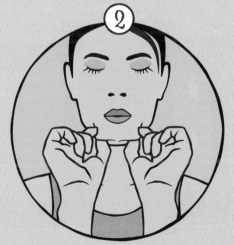

Repeat the action at intervals along the jawline.

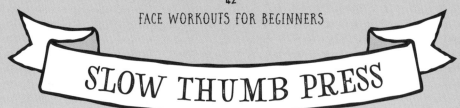

SLOW THUMB PRESS

Applying slow pressure along the jawline, from the chin to the ears, increases blood flow in the area. The activation of the small muscles under the jawbone improves circulation as fluid moves and unblocks nodules of tension.

Benefits

Immediate reduction of fluid and tension. Improved quality of skin and definition to the jawline area.

REPEAT
3 times

TIME
Up to 1 minute

ENVIRONMENT
Standing or seated. In front of a mirror. With eyes closed

EQUIPMENT
Facial oil or face cream

NOTES
Do not perform if the area is swollen or tender to touch, or after dental care.

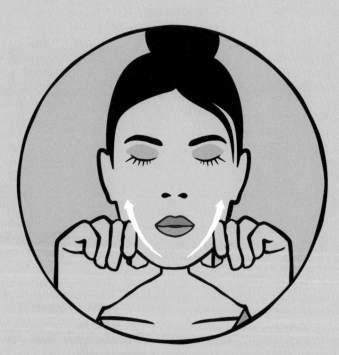

Smooth facial oil or cream over the face and neck. Place the thumbs under the chin and press into the groove between the neck muscles and jawbone, while slowly, continuously, traveling toward the ears.

JAWLINE HOLD

The press-and-hold technique to the jawline brings tender spots to attention. Focusing on your breathing can help if you feel discomfort.

Benefits
Effective toning to the jawline.

REPEAT
Once

TIME
Up to 5 minutes

ENVIRONMENT
Standing or seated.
In front of a mirror.
With eyes closed

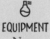
EQUIPMENT
None

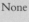
NOTES
Use bent index fingers on the jawline to steady the action. Breathe deeply and steadily throughout.

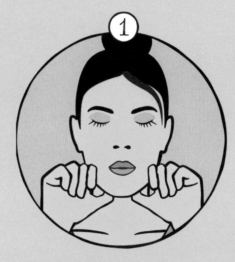

Place the thumbs under the chin and press into the groove between the neck muscles and jawbone. Hold for ten seconds. Breathe through any discomfort to get more relief.

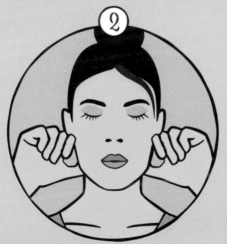

Repeat the action at intervals all along the jawline, working toward the ears.

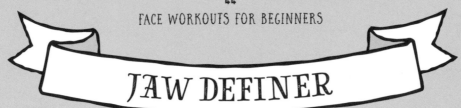

JAW DEFINER

Stretching the neck activates muscles, giving them an efficient workout with optimum results for defining the jaw and reducing the appearance of a double chin.

Benefits
Reduces buildup of fluids around the chin and jawline.

REPEAT
Repeat 8 times. Relax, then repeat another 8 times

TIME
40 seconds

ENVIRONMENT
Standing or seated

EQUIPMENT
None

NOTES
If you feel discomfort in the shoulder or neck, stop immediately. You may find it more comfortable to sit down with the head resting on a cushion for support.

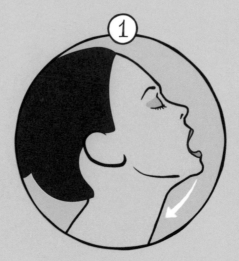

In a comfortable position, tip the head back. Open the mouth and position the jaw forward.

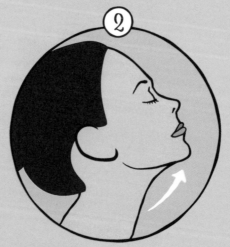

Force the mouth to close. You should feel the stretch around and under the chin.

SLOW JAW DEFINER

By performing a slow version of the Jaw Definer (opposite), the exercise becomes more intense, offering more definition.

Benefits
Reduces buildup of fluids around the chin and jawline.

REPEAT
Open and close 4 times

TIME
Up to 1 minute

ENVIRONMENT
Standing or seated

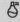
EQUIPMENT
None

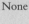
NOTES
If you feel discomfort in the shoulder or neck, stop immediately. You may find it more comfortable to sit down with the head resting on a cushion for support.

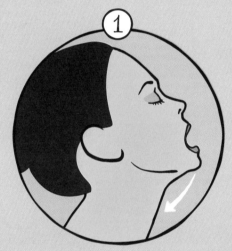

In a comfortable position, tip the head back. Take four seconds to open the mouth and position the jaw forward.

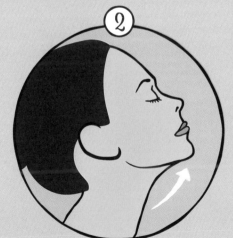

Now take four seconds to close the mouth.

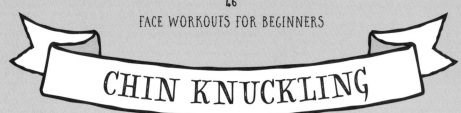

CHIN KNUCKLING

The chin is an area used a lot more than is recognized, and needs attention. This technique of using knuckles provides a deep massage that can cause some discomfort as it works to break down knots.

Benefits

Releases any tensions in the chin area.

REPEAT
Once

TIME
Up to 2 minutes

ENVIRONMENT
Standing or seated

EQUIPMENT
None

NOTES
Do not perform after dental care.

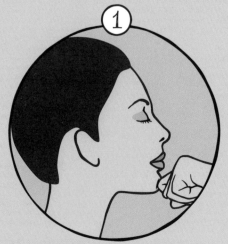

Press the knuckle of one index finger into the center of the chin. Press and hold for ten seconds to adapt to the pressure and sensation.

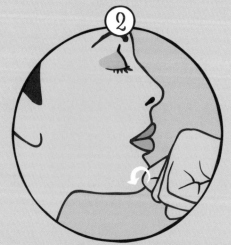

Make tiny circular movements with the knuckle.

CHIN GRIP

Using the press-and-hold technique on the chin releases tension and ensures a complete workout for the jawline.

Benefits

Effectively oxygenates the area and improves movement around the mouth.

REPEAT
Once

TIME
Up to 30 seconds

ENVIRONMENT
Standing or seated

EQUIPMENT
None

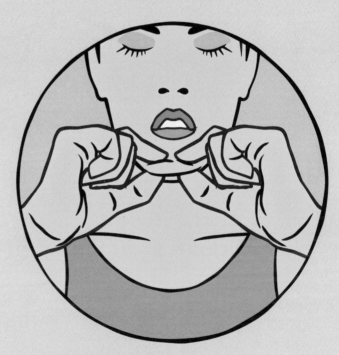

Grip the chin between the index fingers and thumbs, and pull. Hold for up to thirty seconds.

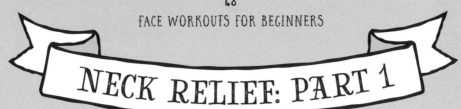

NECK RELIEF: PART 1

The neck often carries a lot of tension, which requires careful and considerate attention through pressure. This exercise provides a sense of centering as well as relieving neck muscles.

Benefits

Instant relief from neck tension. State of relaxation.

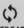

REPEAT
5 times

TIME
15 seconds

ENVIRONMENT
Standing or seated. In front of a mirror. With eyes closed

EQUIPMENT
Facial oil or face cream

NOTES
Ensure shoulders are rolled back and down. Take long, deep breaths.

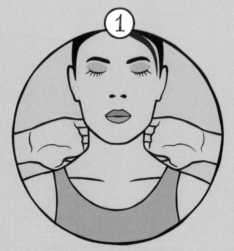

Smooth facial oil or cream over the neck. Position closed fingers at the nape of neck.

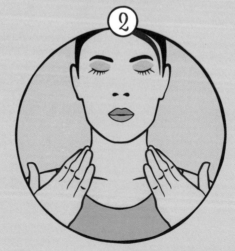

Press firmly as you move down to the collarbone in one continuous movement.

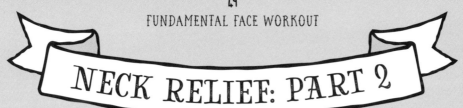

NECK RELIEF: PART 2

This exercise concentrates on relieving a part of the neck that can suffer from unwanted twinges.

Benefits
Instant relief and state of relaxation.

REPEAT
5 times

TIME
15 seconds

ENVIRONMENT
Standing or seated.
In front of a mirror.
With eyes closed

EQUIPMENT
Facial oil or face cream

NOTES
Ensure shoulders are
rolled back and down.
Take long, deep breaths.

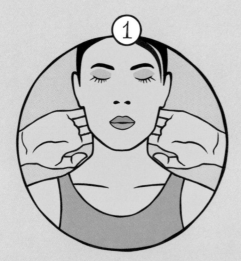

Smooth facial oil or cream over the neck. Place closed fingers behind each ear.

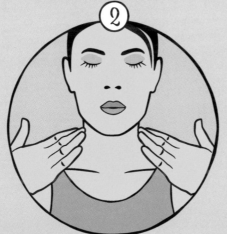

Press down firmly to the base of the neck.

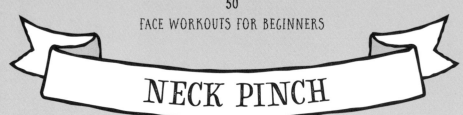

NECK PINCH

The pinch-and-hold technique is effective for creating blood flow and easing tightness in parts of the neck that suffer from strain.

Benefits

Immediate relief from tightness or strain. Over time the exercise can improve definition.

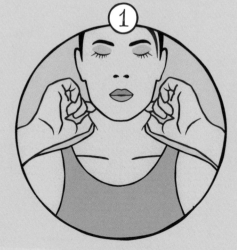

Pinch the skin under the ears between the thumbs and bent index fingers. Hold for twenty seconds or until there is relief.

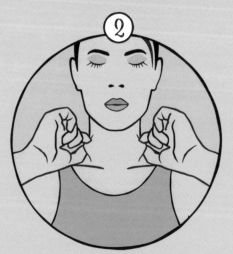

Repeat the pinch action at intervals, working down to the base of the neck.

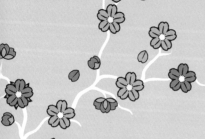

REPEAT
Once

TIME
5 minutes

ENVIRONMENT
Seated

EQUIPMENT
None

NOTES
Do not perform if
under medical care:
This exercise is
performed close to
lymph glands and can
be too sensitive an
exercise to perform if
taking medication.

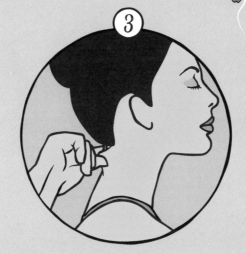

Repeat the same
pinching action,
this time starting
at the nape of the
neck and working
down to the base.

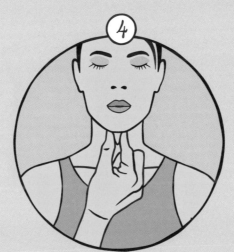

Using one hand,
pinch and hold the
skin under the
chin. Repeat at
intervals, working
down to the chest.

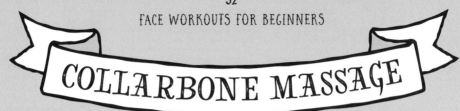

COLLARBONE MASSAGE

With the use of gentle pressure, fluid retention can be moved and toxins reduced. This soothing massage is a powerful self-care practice.

Benefits

De-puffs skin offering definition. Improves circulation and immunity function.

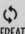

REPEAT
5 times along the collarbone, 5 times under it

TIME
30 seconds

ENVIRONMENT
Standing or seated

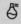

EQUIPMENT
None

NOTES
These massages can be performed on both sides at the same time by crossing the hands over the body.

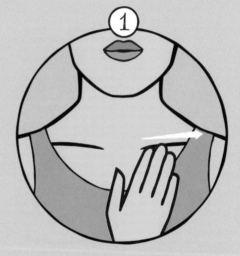

Using flat, closed fingers, gently press along the collarbone, from the inside out toward the shoulder. Repeat four times.

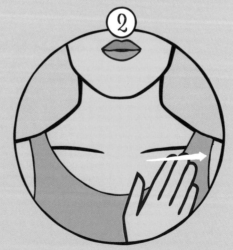

Using flat, closed fingers, gently press under the collarbone four times. Repeat along and under the collarbone on the other side of the body.

EAR TUGGING

Introducing manipulation of the ears as part of a routine activates the lymph nodes and relieves tension in an often-overlooked area.

Benefits

Instant tension reliever. Helps to tone and de-puff the upper jaw.

REPEAT
Twice

TIME
25 seconds

ENVIRONMENT
Standing or seated

EQUIPMENT
None

NOTES
Do not perform if you have a cold or cough, or any ear, nose, or throat issues.

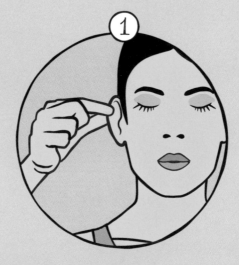

Hold the tops of the ears between the index fingers and thumbs. Pinch and give the ears a tug—a quick pull and release.

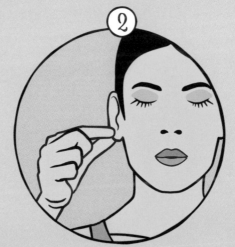

Repeat at regular intervals, working down the outer edge of both ears.

EAR SCRUNCH

Scrunching the ears relieves tension in parts of the ear that are not usually manipulated, offering blood flow and a sense of calm.

Benefits

Instant tension reliever. Helps to tone and de-puff the upper jaw.

REPEAT
5 times. At each repeat change the hand positions slightly to scrunch the ears in different ways

TIME
Up to 1 minute

ENVIRONMENT
Standing or seated

EQUIPMENT
None

NOTES
Do not perform if you have a cold or cough, or any ear, nose, or throat issues.

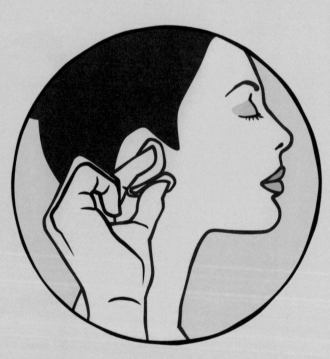

Hold around the edges of the ears with the thumbs and fingertips, and scrunch up the ears. Hold for five seconds.

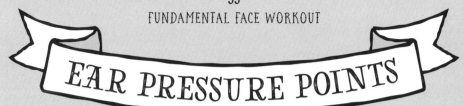

EAR PRESSURE POINTS

The press-and-hold technique stimulates the ears' meridians so that blood flow is activated to sensitive and often tender parts of the outer ear.

Benefits

Offers instant relief.
Softens jawline.
Produces a sense
of well-being.

REPEAT
Once

TIME
Up to 1 minute

ENVIRONMENT
Standing or seated

EQUIPMENT
None

NOTES
Do not perform if you
have a cold or cough,
or any ear, nose, or
throat issues.

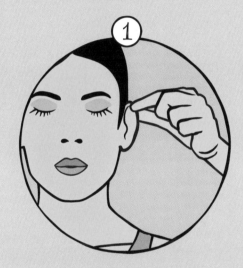

Pinch the tops of the ears between the index fingers and thumbs. Hold for ten seconds.

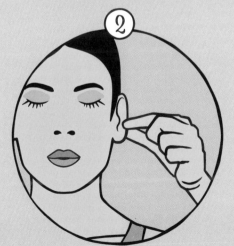

Repeat at intervals all the way down the outer edge of both ears.

MOUTH IN MOTION

THIS CHAPTER OFFERS EFFICIENT TECHNIQUES—BOTH
EXTERNAL AND INTERNAL—TO HELP PREVENT SYMPTOMS
SUCH AS SAGGING, A DOWN-TURNED MOUTH, AND TRAUMA
LINES. BE PREPARED FOR AN INTENSE WORKOUT!

START THIS SERIES OF EXERCISES WITH
DEEP BREATHS (SEE PAGE 16).

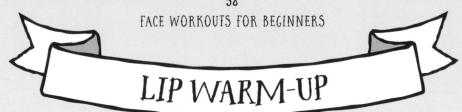

LIP WARM-UP

A quick lip warm-up keeps the mouth—usually a much-overworked part of the face—relaxed.

Benefits
Instantly loosens tension in the lips.

REPEAT
10 times, building to vibration of the lips

TIME
20 seconds

ENVIRONMENT
Standing or seated

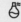

EQUIPMENT
None

NOTES
As more vibration and sound is created on each exhale, more relaxation is achieved.

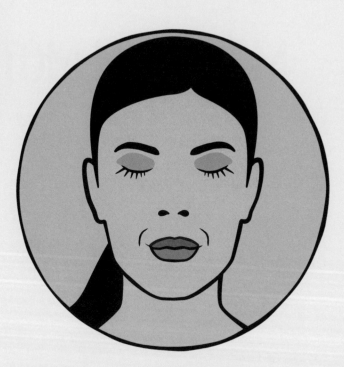

Gently blow through the lips while keeping the mouth rested. Gradually build up the effort to try to create a vibration and sound.

INFLATED CHEEKS

Activating the muscles around the mouth, where deep lines are often set, can help improve mobility.

Benefits

Targets signs of stress and tension around the mouth, and premature aging.

REPEAT
Twice

TIME
1 minute

ENVIRONMENT
Standing or seated

EQUIPMENT
None

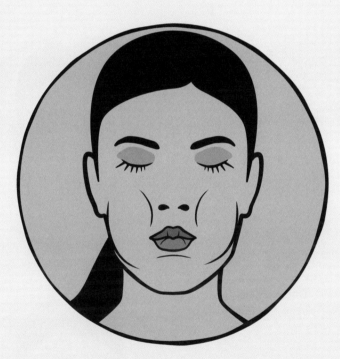

Inflate the cheeks fully with air and hold for ten seconds. Release. Inflate the cheeks fully with air and hold for twenty seconds.

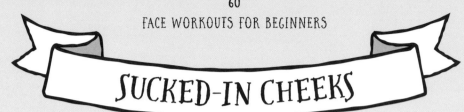

SUCKED-IN CHEEKS

This exercise is deeply intense, enough to tone the area worked over time. As the muscles become activated, uneven tension is loosened.

Benefits
Effective toning. Defines cheekbones and relieves tension in the lower cheek area.

REPEAT
Twice

TIME
Up to 30 seconds

ENVIRONMENT
Standing or seated. In front of a mirror

EQUIPMENT
None

NOTES
Over time, build up to a repeat of 4 times, or holding for 20 to 30 seconds.

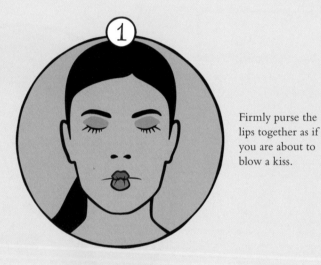

Firmly purse the lips together as if you are about to blow a kiss.

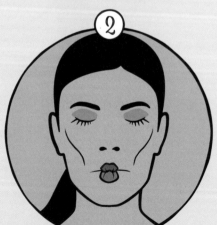

Suck in both cheeks, then force more suction so that the cheeks are entirely deflated with the lips sucked inward. Hold for fifteen seconds.

CHEEK PUSHING

Working from the inside of the mouth is a practical and powerful
way to rouse tense muscles and promote toning.

Benefits
Immense relief.
Increased mobility
and toning to the
facial structure.

REPEAT
Twice on each side
of the mouth

TIME
Up to 3 minutes

ENVIRONMENT
Standing or seated.
In front of a mirror

EQUIPMENT
None

NOTES
This is an ideal exercise
post-recovery or
post-trauma. Do
not perform straight
after dental work.

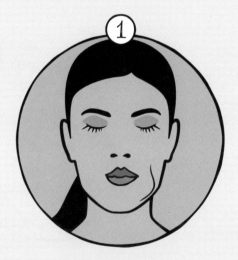

Push the tongue
into the side of the
cheek as firmly as
possible and hold
for a few seconds.

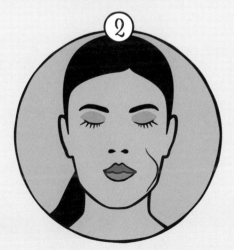

Maneuver the
tongue around the
cheek areas and
hold for a few
seconds or until
tension is released.
Try to push the
tongue into hard-
to-reach areas.
Repeat with the
other cheek.

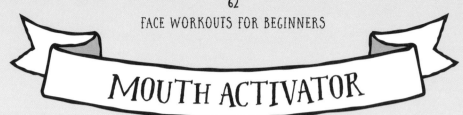

MOUTH ACTIVATOR

This intense workout to the lips and mouth area efficiently energizes, while strengthening the framework of the lower part of the face.

Benefits

Tones and defines around the lips, mouth, and cheeks.

REPEAT
Twice

TIME
Up to 30 seconds

ENVIRONMENT
Standing or seated

EQUIPMENT
None

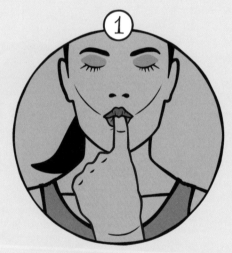

Purse the lips firmly together with the index finger placed between them. Use the lips to move the finger forward and backward.

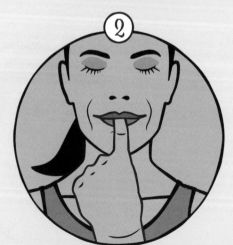

Continue for up to fifteen seconds.

LIP PUSHING

Concentrating on the small features, such as the lips, can profoundly tone the area all around them.

Benefits

Targets and prevents a downturned mouth and sagging. Increased mobility.

REPEAT
4 times

TIME
Up to 1 minute

ENVIRONMENT
None

EQUIPMENT
Standing or seated

NOTES
Do not perform this exercise if you have had recent dental work.

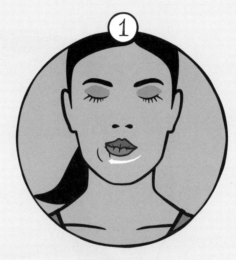

① Push the tongue below the lower lip and sweep along from one side to the other. Hold for ten seconds at the lip edge.

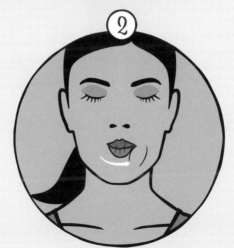

② Sweep the tongue back to the other side and hold for ten seconds at that lip edge.

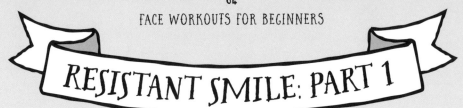

RESISTANT SMILE: PART 1

Creating resistance during this exercise makes the muscles work
harder and encourages firming and toning around the mouth.

Benefits

Tackles deep lines
and sagging while
relieving tension
around the mouth.

REPEAT
5 times

TIME
Up to 30 seconds

ENVIRONMENT
Standing or seated.
In front of a mirror

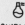

EQUIPMENT
None

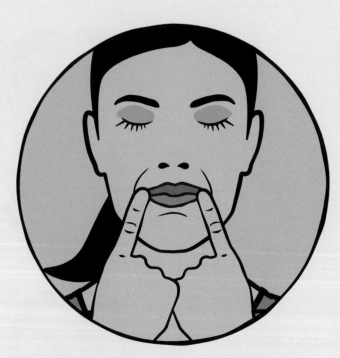

Relax the face and mouth. Press the index fingers firmly
on the corners of the mouth to create tension, then force
a smile, all the while using the fingers to resist the smile.
Hold for five seconds.

RESISTANT SMILE: PART 2

This exercise creates resistance in reverse, ensuring all mouth muscles are activated to achieve the best toning results.

Benefits
Tackles deep lines and prevents sagging around the mouth.

REPEAT
5 times

TIME
Up to 30 seconds

ENVIRONMENT
Standing or seated. In front of a mirror

EQUIPMENT
None

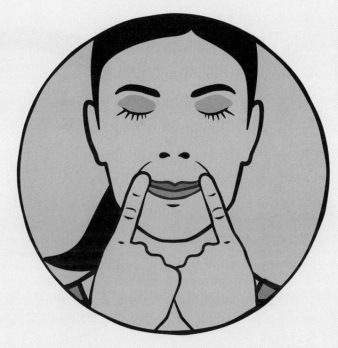

Smile and press the index fingers firmly on the corners of the mouth. Try to force the lips to purse together while using the index fingers to resist the effort. Hold for five seconds.

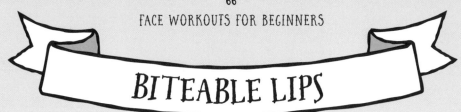

BITEABLE LIPS

Intense pressure to the lips offers relief and increased mobility,
but also encourages blood flow to energize the area.

Benefits

Gives an instant
lip-plumping effect.

REPEAT
10 times or until
tension is released

TIME
Up to 1 minute

ENVIRONMENT
Standing or seated.
In front of a mirror

EQUIPMENT
With or without
lip balm

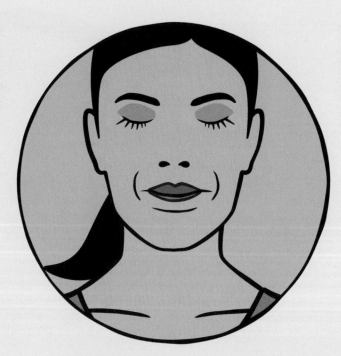

Motion the lips into the mouth while adding pressure,
using the teeth to increase intensity as you bring the
lips back to resting.

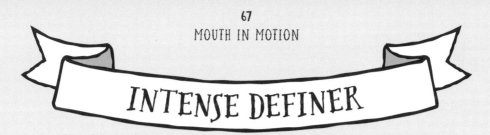

INTENSE DEFINER

Knuckling deeply around the mouth slowly offers effective results to where trauma lines occur. This is also a helpful way to avoid deep lines.

Benefits
Instant relief. Softens deep lines.

REPEAT
5 times

TIME
Up to 2 minutes

ENVIRONMENT
Standing or seated. In front of a mirror

EQUIPMENT
None

NOTES
Not advisable after dental work.

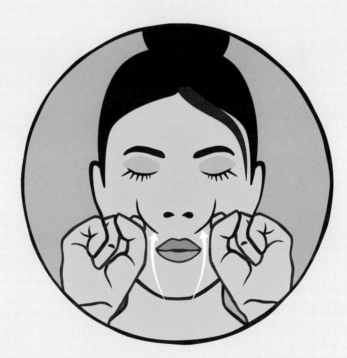

Place the knuckles of the index fingers to the sides of the chin. Slowly travel up the side of the mouth just before reaching the nostrils, then hold for five seconds.

WARNING

No immense or shooting pain should be experienced during any of these exercises. Should this occur, seek medical advice.

5

SCULPTED CHEEKS

THIS INTENSE WORKOUT PRESENTS A DYNAMIC GUIDE TO
SCULPTING THE CHEEKS USING SLOW AND STEADY MOTIONS,
OFFERING OPTIMUM RESULTS TO TONE AND DEFINE THE AREA.

BEGIN THIS WORKOUT WITH DEEP BREATHS
(SEE PAGE 16).

NASAL PASSAGE PRESS

Sensitive pressure points inform the body of blockages and a buildup of tension. The oxygenation that occurs with the press-and-hold technique works to unblock the area.

Benefits
Instant relief.
Plumpness to cheeks.

REPEAT
Twice

TIME
Up to 45 seconds

ENVIRONMENT
Standing or seated.
In front of a mirror

EQUIPMENT
None

NOTES
Breathe through the
hold position.

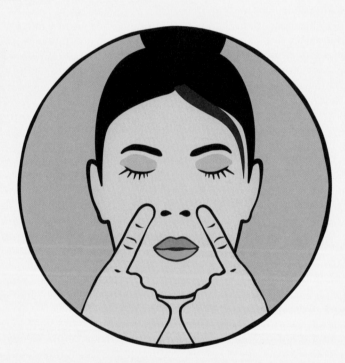

Place the index fingers beside the nasal passage. Press and hold firmly for twenty seconds.

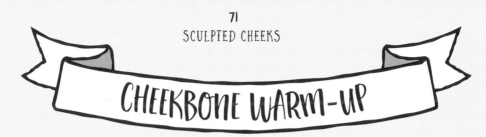

CHEEKBONE WARM-UP

A great deal of tension is unknowingly built up under the cheekbones. Over time tautness in the area denies facial muscle mobility, resulting in puffiness and deep lines.

Benefits
Activates blood flow. Releases tightness to promote toning.

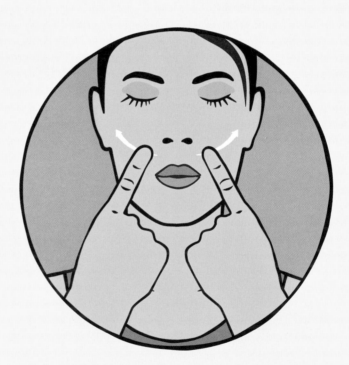

REPEAT
5 times

TIME
Up to 1 minute

ENVIRONMENT
Standing or seated. In front of a mirror

EQUIPMENT
Facial oil or face cream

NOTES
Breathe through the pressure.

Smooth facial oil or cream over the face. Start by placing the index fingers beside the nasal passages. Press firmly under the cheekbones and move slowly along to the ears.

CHEEKBONE KNUCKLING

Using the knuckles to get to hard-to-reach areas of the face
is effective for promoting oxygenation to help disperse fluid
that causes puffiness.

Benefits

Releases knots for
immediate relief.
Promotes contoured
cheeks.

REPEAT

5 times, taking a short
break before repeating

TIME

Up to 2 minutes

ENVIRONMENT

Standing or seated.
In front of a mirror

EQUIPMENT

Facial oil or face cream

NOTES

Breathe through
the pressure.

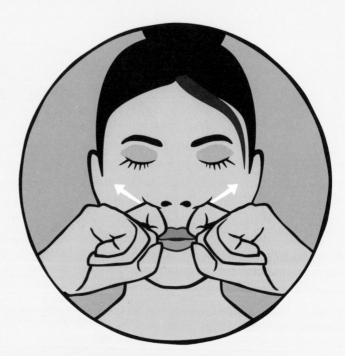

Smooth facial oil or cream over the face. Press the
knuckles of the index fingers beside the nasal passages.
Press firmly under the cheekbones and glide, slowly
and steadily, to the ears.

CHEEKBONE DEFINER: PART 1

The press-and-hold technique offers further definition as well as oxygenation, and alleviates muscular tension on a deeper level.

Benefits
Remarkable relief and instant sculpting effect to cheeks.

REPEAT
Once

TIME
Up to 2 minutes

ENVIRONMENT
Standing or seated. In front of a mirror

EQUIPMENT
Facial oil or face cream

NOTES
It is essential that you breathe through the 5-second hold.

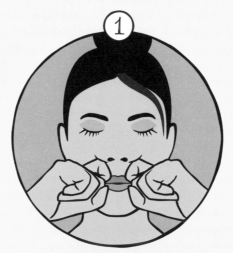

Apply facial oil or cream to the face. Press the knuckles of the index fingers beside the nasal passages and hold firmly for five seconds.

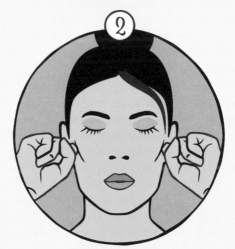

Repeat the action at intervals along and under the cheekbones until you reach the base of the ears.

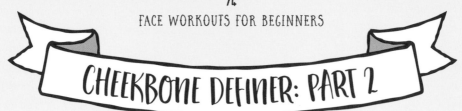

CHEEKBONE DEFINER: PART 2

This exercise concentrates further intensity to the contours of the cheeks, focusing on harder-to-reach areas.

Benefits
Remarkable relief and instant sculpting effect to the bone structure.

REPEAT
Once

TIME
Up to 5 minutes

ENVIRONMENT
Standing or seated. In front of a mirror

EQUIPMENT
Facial oil or face cream

NOTES
It is essential that you breathe through the 5-second hold and the downward movement.

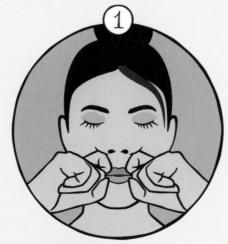

Smooth facial oil or cream over the face. Press the knuckles of the index fingers beside the nasal passages and hold firmly for five seconds.

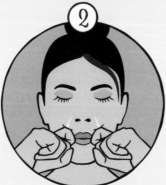

Slowly, and with pressure, move the knuckles downward into the hollows of the cheeks.

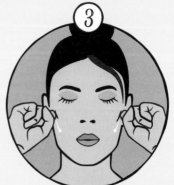

Repeat Steps 1 and 2 at intervals, working along and under the cheekbones until you reach the base of the ears.

CHEEKBONE DEFINER: PART 3

By adding an additional movement to this sequence of exercises the sensations are intensified, as are the remarkable results.

Benefits
Remarkable relief and instant sculpting effect to the bone structure.

REPEAT
Once

TIME
Up to 5 minutes

ENVIRONMENT
Standing or seated. In front of a mirror

EQUIPMENT
Facial oil or face cream

NOTES
It is essential that you breathe through the 5-second hold and the downward movement.

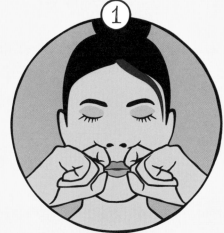

Apply facial oil or cream to the face. Press the knuckles of the index fingers beside the nasal passages and hold firmly for five seconds.

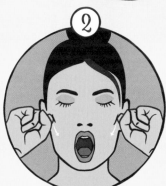

Slowly, and with pressure, move the knuckles downward into the hollows of the cheeks while opening the mouth.

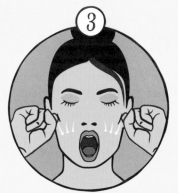

Repeat Steps 1 and 2 at intervals, working along and under the cheekbones until you reach the base of the ears.

KNUCKLE HOLD

This exercise intensely activates the area under the cheekbones to target and relieve tension and define the cheekbones and facial structure.

Benefits
Relief to deep framework of facial muscles and noticeable definition.

REPEAT
Open and close mouth 10 times

TIME
Up to 1 minute

ENVIRONMENT
Seated

EQUIPMENT
Facial oil or face cream

NOTES
For deep and more even pressure, you can lean your elbows on a table with eyes closed. Do not forget to breathe deeply.

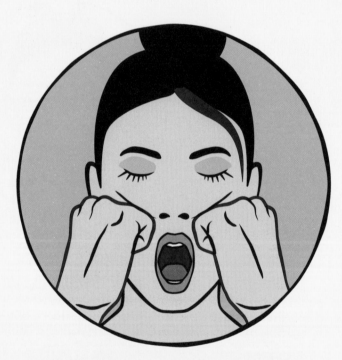

Smooth facial oil or cream over the face. With the hands in a fist, place the knuckles as deeply and firmly as possible under the cheekbones. Very slowly, open and close the mouth.

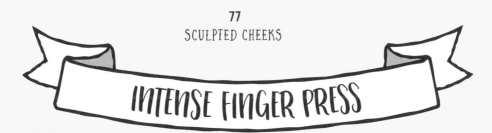

INTENSE FINGER PRESS

Pressing and holding close to the jaw joint offers deep relief to an area prone to carrying stress and becoming stiff, which often means the cheekbones become less defined over time.

Benefits
Redefines bone structure while offering intense relief.

REPEAT
10 times

TIME
Up to 1 minute

ENVIRONMENT
Seated

EQUIPMENT
None

NOTES
For deep and more even pressure, lean the elbows on a table with eyes closed. Do not forget to breathe deeply. This exercise is not recommended after dental treatment.

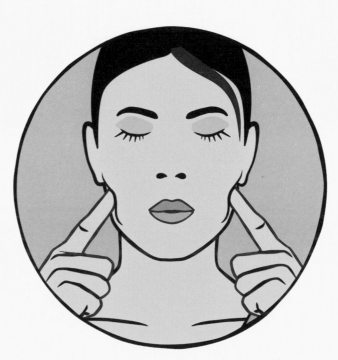

Press the index fingers firmly into the dip close to the jaw joints and hold for ten seconds.

CHEEKBONE THUMB PRESS

Manipulating areas in an upward motion encourages fluid to disperse
and de-puffing to take place.

Benefits

Definition to bone
structure and
reduction of tension.

REPEAT
Once

TIME
Up to 1 minute

ENVIRONMENT
Standing or seated.
In front of a mirror

EQUIPMENT
Facial oil or face cream

NOTES
Breathe through the
10-second hold.

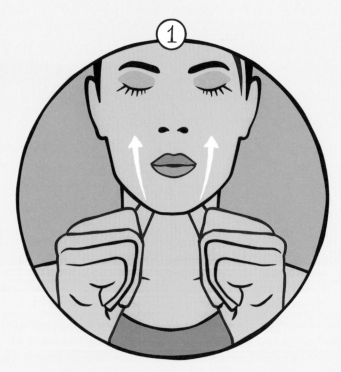

Apply facial oil or cream to the face. Press and glide the
thumbs from the chin directly up to the cheekbones, and
hold for ten seconds.

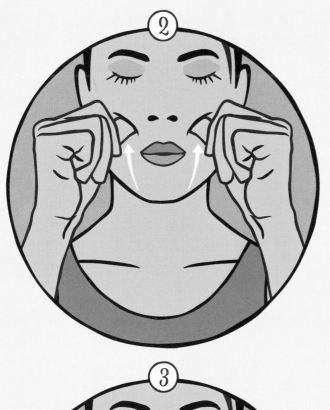

Repeat the action from the chin to a roughly adjacent area along the cheekbone.

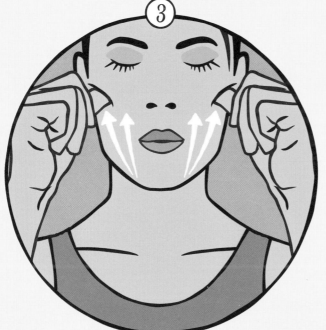

Continue the action from the chin at intervals along the cheekbone until you reach the end of the cheek hollows.

WARNING

No immense or shooting pain should be experienced during any of these exercises. Should this occur, seek medical advice.

FOREHEAD FOCUS

THE FOREHEAD REQUIRES MUCH ATTENTION IN ORDER TO
AVOID OR LESSEN HORIZONTAL AND FROWN LINES, USUALLY
BY EMPLOYING SMOOTH MOTIONS USING THE EYEBROWS AS
A GUIDE. WITH THE USE OF A FACIAL OIL OR FACE CREAM,
THESE EXERCISES IMPROVE SKIN QUALITY, CAN SOFTEN
LINES, AND SOOTHE TENSION HEADACHES, ESPECIALLY
AROUND THE DELICATE CURVES OF THE TEMPLES. IN
ADDITION, THEY OFFER AN AWARENESS OF FROWNING AND
CAN HELP YOU MOVE AWAY FROM SUCH HABITS.

START THIS SERIES OF EXERCISES WITH
DEEP BREATHS (SEE PAGE 16).

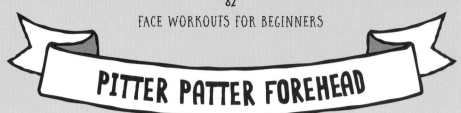

PITTER PATTER FOREHEAD

Stimulating the forehead with the tips of the fingers is an effective way to warm up the area.

Benefits
Warms up and soothes the area.

REPEAT
Once

TIME
30 seconds

ENVIRONMENT
Standing or seated

EQUIPMENT
None

NOTES
Avoid the temples.

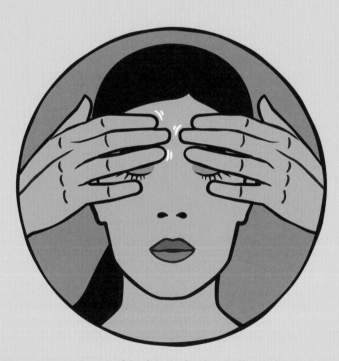

Using the tips of the fingers, firmly tap all over the forehead, alternating fingers while tapping.

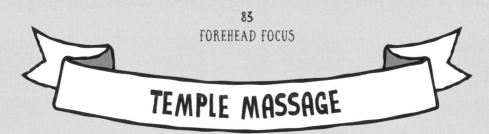

TEMPLE MASSAGE

The delicate temple areas tend to carry tension that requires attention using careful techniques.

Benefits
Instant release of tension.

REPEAT
10 times forward,
10 times back

TIME
Approximately
20 seconds

ENVIRONMENT
Standing or seated

EQUIPMENT
None

NOTES
Never apply firm pressure to the temples.

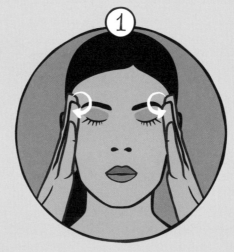

Close the fingers together and place flat fingertips on the temples. Use gentle pressure to massage in a circular motion. Circle forward ten times.

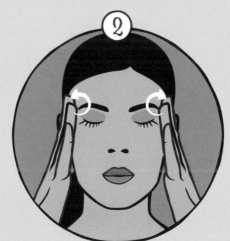

Repeat ten times in a backward motion.

UPWARD MASSAGE

Manipulating the skin upward encourages the forehead to remain smooth and to avoid frowning.

Benefits
Helps to soften horizontal and vertical lines.

REPEAT
5 times

TIME
Up to 1 minute

ENVIRONMENT
Standing or seated.
In front of a mirror

EQUIPMENT
Facial oil or face cream

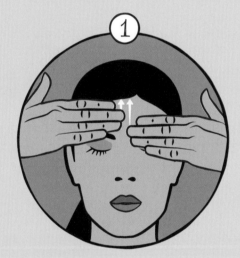

Smooth facial oil or cream onto the fingers. Close the fingers together and place flat fingertips on the center of the forehead. With firm pressure, sweep upward while alternating the hands.

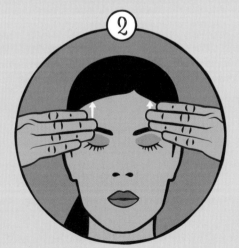

Continue this action while working outward from the center.

CENTRAL MASSAGE

Massaging one specific area, such the central part of the forehead, releases an immense amount of tension and helps to reawaken a state of well-being.

Benefits
Can relieve tension headaches and center the mind.

REPEAT
Once, or up to 3 times for tension headaches

TIME
20 seconds at a time

ENVIRONMENT
Standing or seated

EQUIPMENT
None

NOTES
Can be performed with the elbows resting on a table for comfort.

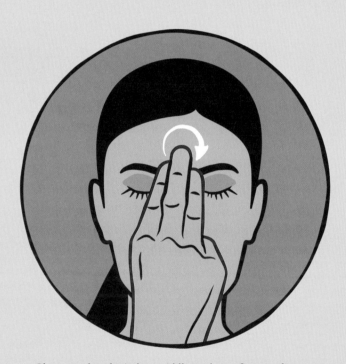

Close together the index, middle, and ring fingers of one hand and place on the center of the forehead. Using firm pressure, move the fingertips in a small circular motion for twenty seconds.

BROW PRESS

Once some tension is released along the brows there is increased mobility with less chance of the forehead becoming overused.

Benefits
Instant relief and increased mobility.

🔄
REPEAT
10 times

⏱
TIME
Approximately
1 minute

🪑
ENVIRONMENT
Standing or seated

⚗
EQUIPMENT
None

📌
NOTES
The exercise can be more relaxing if performed with the eyes closed.

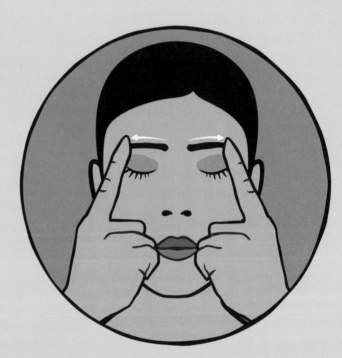

Using the index fingers, press firmly onto the inner brows, then continue to press very slowly along the length of the brows.

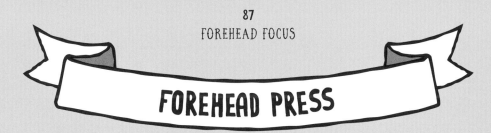

FOREHEAD PRESS

Using fluid movements over the forehead can offer much relief and encourage blood flow and a softened surface.

Benefits
Instantly relieves tension, smooths skin, and can soften horizontal lines.

REPEAT
10 times

TIME
Up to 1 minute

ENVIRONMENT
Standing or seated. In front of a mirror

EQUIPMENT
Facial oil or face cream

NOTES
Make sure you work in one continuous movement.

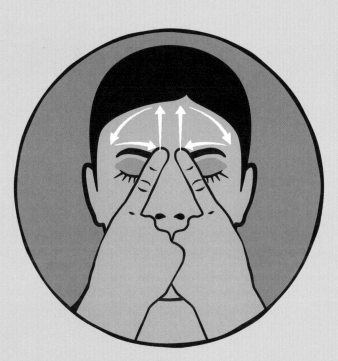

Apply a small amount of facial oil or cream to the forehead. Press the index fingers onto the inner brows, then, in one movement, press firmly up to the hairline, sweep around the circumference of the forehead and back along the brows.

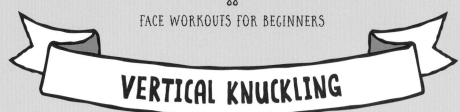

VERTICAL KNUCKLING

Using the knuckles allows for intense pressure that offers profound relief and an increase in oxygenation, leading to reenergized and smoother skin.

Benefits

Instant release of muscular stiffness. Smoother skin. Lessens frown lines and helps to avoid both vertical and horizontal lines.

REPEAT
Once

TIME
Up to 2 minutes

ENVIRONMENT
Standing or seated. In front of a mirror

EQUIPMENT
Facial oil or face cream

NOTES
Do not perform this exercise if you have a migraine or headache.

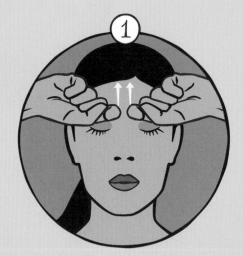

Smooth a little facial oil or cream over the forehead. Place the knuckles of the index fingers between the brows. Pressing firmly, slowly glide the knuckles upward, toward the hairline.

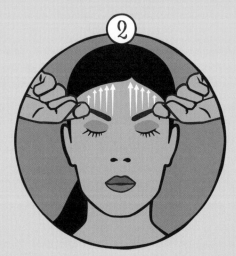

Return to the next area along on the inner brow and again press firmly up to the hairline. Repeat the action at intervals along the brows.

HORIZONTAL KNUCKLING

By knuckling the forehead in a horizontal direction more inactive muscles are activated, leading to a smoother, more refined forehead and increased awareness of how to avoid frowning.

Benefits

Instant release of muscular stiffness. Smoother skin. Lessens frown lines and helps to avoid both vertical and horizontal lines.

REPEAT
Once

TIME
Up to 2 minutes

ENVIRONMENT
Standing or seated. In front of a mirror

EQUIPMENT
Facial oil or face cream

NOTES
Do not perform this exercise if you have a migraine or headache.

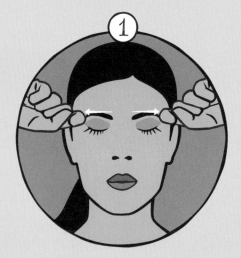

Smooth a little facial oil or cream over the forehead. Place the knuckles of the index fingers between the brows. Pressing firmly, slowly glide the knuckles along the brow-line.

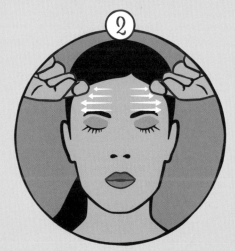

Repeat just above the eyebrows and continue repeating the action at intervals until you reach the hairline, using the brows as a guide each time.

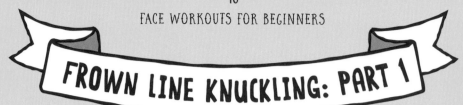

FROWN LINE KNUCKLING: PART 1

Tackling frown lines directly assists in avoiding future lines and brings awareness to how the face sits, since frowning often goes unnoticed until the lines appear.

Benefits

Lessens frown lines and offers instant results. Eases muscles.

REPEAT
Twice

TIME
Up to 1 minute

ENVIRONMENT
Standing or seated.
In front of a mirror

EQUIPMENT
None

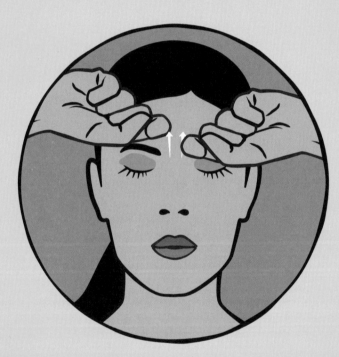

Place the knuckles of the index fingers in between the brows. Press firmly and glide upward in twenty short, quick strokes, alternating between the left and right knuckles.

FROWN LINE KNUCKLING: PART 2

Using a circular motion with the knuckles manipulates and stimulates the muscles more broadly for a smoother surface area.

Benefits
Lessens frown lines and offers instant results. Eases muscles.

REPEAT
Twice

TIME
Up to 1 minute

ENVIRONMENT
Standing or seated. In front of a mirror

EQUIPMENT
None

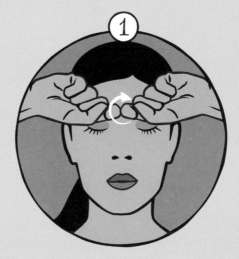

1

Place the knuckles of the index fingers in between the brows. Pressing firmly, make tiny circular motions.

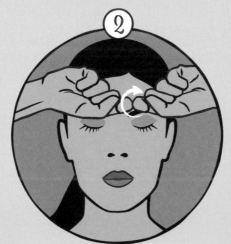

2

Move the motion from close to the inner part of the right brow, back to the center, then to the inner part of the left brow.

NOTES

It is advised that most of these exercises be performed in front of a mirror for accuracy, and that contact lenses be removed.

OPTIC VERVE

THIS CHAPTER CONTAINS THE MOST MINIMAL WORKOUT,
YET MOST EFFECTIVE TECHNIQUES TO REVIVE AND DE-PUFF
THE ORBITAL AREA, AS WELL AS IMPROVE STRENGTH IN THE
MUSCLES TO HELP PREVENT HOODED EYES. WITH EYES BEING
THE MOST DELICATE PART OF THE FACE, IT IS IMPERATIVE
THAT A LIGHT TOUCH IS ADMINISTERED, USING AN
EYE CREAM OR SERUM IF DESIRED.

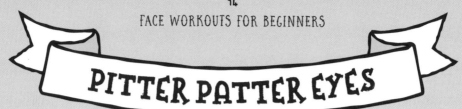

PITTER PATTER EYES

Simple techniques such as "pitter pattering" over closed eyes helps
to wake up and reenergize the area.

Benefits
Revives and gently
massages.

REPEAT
Once

TIME
Up to 1 minute

ENVIRONMENT
Standing or seated.
In front of a mirror

EQUIPMENT
None

NOTES
Can be performed
with the elbows resting
on a table for comfort.

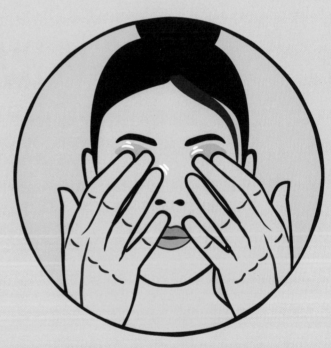

Close the eyes and use the tips of the fingers to gently tap
over the eyelids, alternating fingers while tapping.

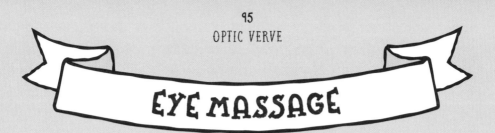

EYE MASSAGE

This exercise is a gentle way to soothe and revive tired eyes.

Benefits
Energizes the eyes.

REPEAT
10 times clockwise,
10 times
counterclockwise

TIME
Up to 1 minute

ENVIRONMENT
Seated

EQUIPMENT
None

NOTES
Can be performed
with the elbows resting
on a table for comfort.

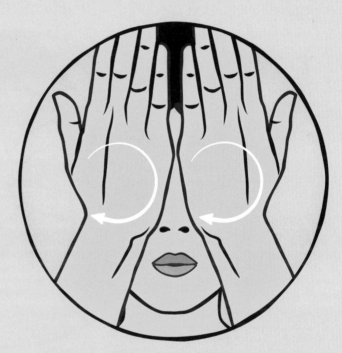

Place both hands over the eyes, with the curve of the palm over the eyes so it doesn't touch them. Use the pads at the top of the palms to press gently on the orbital bone above the eyes, making slow, circular motions. Make ten circles in a clockwise direction. Repeat in a counterclockwise direction.

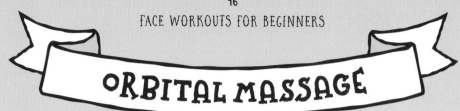

ORBITAL MASSAGE

Massaging the orbital bone helps eyes to feel more awake,
and to disperse fluid that builds up under the eyes.

Benefits
Instantly energizes
and de-puffs the eyes.

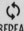

REPEAT
Once

TIME
2 minutes

ENVIRONMENT
Standing or seated

EQUIPMENT
None

NOTES
Best performed slowly.

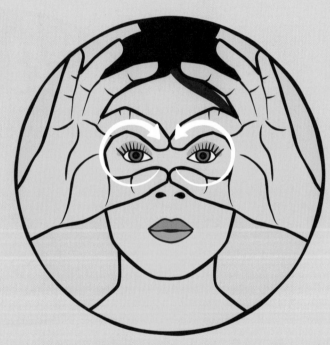

Make the index fingers and thumbs into two "C" shapes
and place them on the orbital bone around the eyes. With
firm pressure make slow, circular motions, using the
thumbs and index fingers to massage all over the bone.

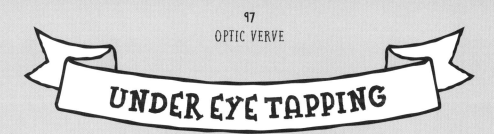

UNDER EYE TAPPING

Another effective way to move fluid around the eyes and create the sensation of awakening them is by tapping on the delicate part around the eye.

Benefits
De-puffs and de-stresses the areas around the eyes.

REPEAT
5 times

TIME
2 minutes

ENVIRONMENT
Standing or seated

EQUIPMENT
None

Using the ring fingers, start close to the bridge of the nose and firmly tap underneath the eye, moving along to the outer eye.

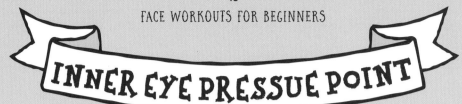

INNER EYE PRESSUE POINT

Pressure on specific areas helps banish tension, unblock stress, and force balance.

Benefits

Helps to de-puff around the eyes, improving eye contours. Offers instant relief for tension headaches and eye strain.

REPEAT

Press and hold for 10 seconds, or until there is relief.

TIME

10 seconds

ENVIRONMENT

Standing or seated

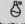

EQUIPMENT

None

NOTES

Take deep, steady breaths. Hands can be unclasped also.

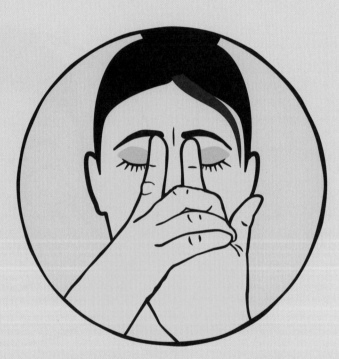

Place the index fingers just under each inner brow bone with clasped hands for even pressure. Find the tender spot, then press firmly and hold.

BROW PUSH-UPS

Resisting muscle movement is an impressive way to strengthen underused muscles around the eyes, which can become hooded.

Benefits
Direct strengthening to the upper eyes.

REPEAT
10 times

TIME
Up to 1 minute

ENVIRONMENT
Standing or seated

EQUIPMENT
None

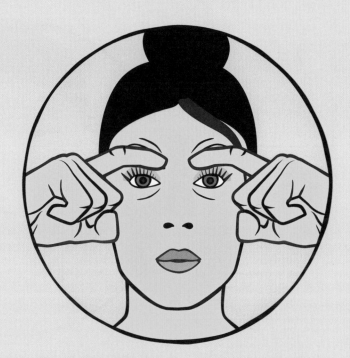

Place the outsides of the index fingers on the eyebrows. Press down firmly while attempting to frown for five seconds, using the fingers to try to resist the movement.

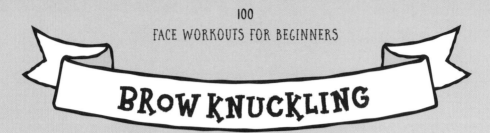

BROW KNUCKLING

Knuckling under the eyebrows helps to define the contours of
the eyes and avoid hooding.

Benefits

Helps to lift brows
to promote a wide-
awake effect.

REPEAT
5 times

TIME
Up to 1 minute

ENVIRONMENT
Standing or seated.
In front of a mirror

EQUIPMENT
None

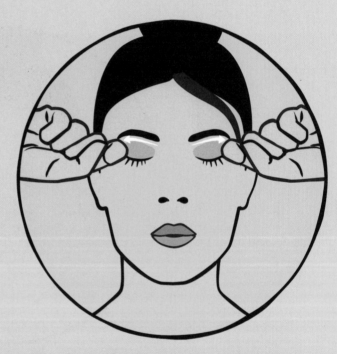

Place the knuckles of the index fingers under the inner
brows. Use a firm stroke to pull the knuckles under and
along the length of the brows.

INTENSE UNDER EYE MASSAGE

Pulling the skin away from the eyes allows for a deeper, more precise massage to the hollow areas under the eyes.

Benefits
Instantly de-puffs around the eyes.

REPEAT
Twice on both sides

TIME
Approximately 2 minutes

ENVIRONMENT
Standing or seated. In front of a mirror

EQUIPMENT
None

NOTES
Do not apply heavy pressure to this area.

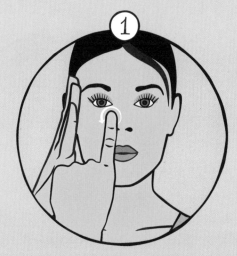

Gently pull away the skin on the outer part of the eye and hold in place. Use the index finger of the other hand to massage under the eye in a gentle, circular motion starting near the bridge of the nose.

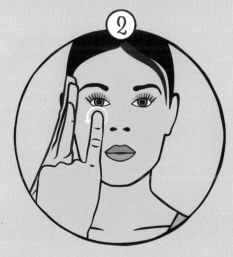

Repeat the action at intervals along the area under the eye until you reach the outer edge. Repeat on other side.

UNDER EYE SWEEP

The sweeping motion in this exercise emphasizes the importance of dispersing fluid from under the eyes to reveal a well-rested look.

Benefits
Instantly de-puffs around the eyes and defines contours.

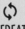

REPEAT
Twice on both sides

TIME
Approximately 1 minute

ENVIRONMENT
Standing or seated. In front of a mirror

EQUIPMENT
None

NOTES
Do not apply heavy pressure to this area.

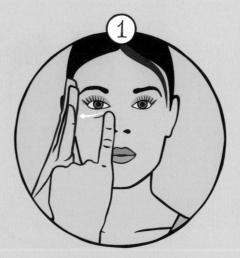

Gently pull away the skin on the outer part of the eye and hold in place. Use the index finger of the other hand to gently sweep under the eye, starting near the bridge of the nose and sweeping to the outer edge. Repeat seven more times.

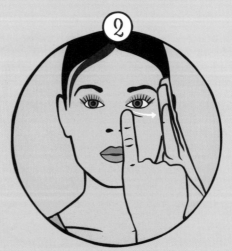

Repeat to make eight sweeps on the other side.

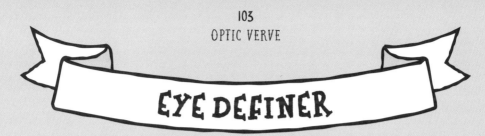

EYE DEFINER

This exercise demonstrates that the delicate skin around the eyes can be carefully exercised using very little manipulation and pressure.

Benefits

Helps flatten and de-puff under the eyes.

REPEAT
10 times on each eye

TIME
Up to 30 seconds

ENVIRONMENT
Standing or seated. In front of a mirror

EQUIPMENT
None

NOTES
Not advisable after eye surgery or eye procedures.

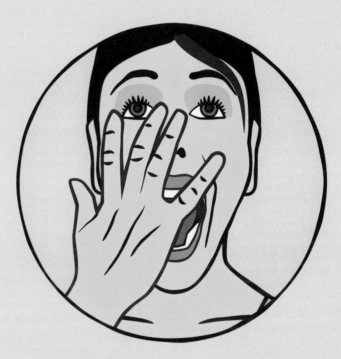

Place the middle finger on the inner eye with the index finger on the outer edge. Pressing firmly, look upward without creasing the forehead and make an "O" shape with the mouth. There should be a slight pull around the eyes. Hold for a few seconds, release, and repeat ten times. Repeat on the other eye.

NOTES

It is advised that most of these exercises
be performed in front of a mirror for
accuracy in locating each facial zone.

SKIN ILLUMINATION WORKOUT

THIS SERIES OF EXERCISES FOCUSES ON REVIVING SKIN
USING SWEEPING MOTIONS TO FLUSH TOXINS, AND THE
PINCH-AND-HOLD TECHNIQUE TO PROMOTE BLOOD FLOW AND
REVEAL A MORE RADIANT COMPLEXION. THE PINCH OFFERS
INTENSE RELIEF IN A FIVE-SECOND HOLD, WHICH IS WHY IT
IS ADVISABLE TO USE A FAVORITE SCENTED FACIAL OIL OR
FACE CREAM TO HELP YOU BREATHE THROUGH EACH HOLD.

START THIS SERIES OF EXERCISES
WITH DEEP BREATHS WITH SCENT
(SEE PAGE 17).

LIGHT FACIAL MASSAGE

This exercise helps to create a balanced state of mind and gently wakes up the face.

Benefits

Gentle awakening technique to apply facial oil or face cream, which can be performed daily.

REPEAT
Once

TIME
15 seconds

ENVIRONMENT
Standing or seated. In front of a mirror

EQUIPMENT
Scented facial oil or face cream

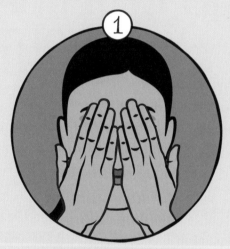

Apply scented facial oil or cream to the palms of the hands and press together. Pat the palms on the face, while deeply inhaling the scent.

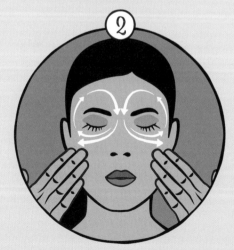

Using light pressure, glide the hands outward over the cheeks, then over the forehead, down the nose, and over the cheeks to the ears.

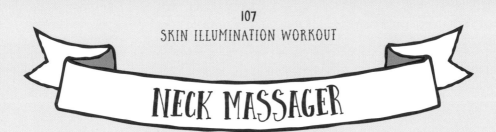

SKIN ILLUMINATION WORKOUT

NECK MASSAGER

An effective way to move fluid retention is through massage, which
will also stimulate the lymph glands into oxygenating.

Benefits
Promotes definition
on the neck and chin.

REPEAT
Perform massage strokes
20 times

TIME
Up to 1 minute

ENVIRONMENT
Standing or seated.
In front of a mirror

EQUIPMENT
Scented facial oil
or face cream

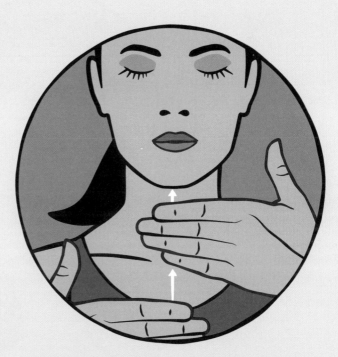

Apply a little scented facial oil or cream to the fingertips,
then smooth it through the fingers. With closed fingers at
the base of the neck, lightly stroke up to the chin,
making sure to alternate hands.

COLLARBONE PRESS

With the use of firm pressure, fluid retention can be effectively moved, reducing toxins and increasing blood flow.

Benefits

De-puffs the skin, offering definition to the décolletage area. Improves circulation to benefit skin's clarity.

REPEAT
Once

TIME
Approximately 3 minutes

ENVIRONMENT
Standing or seated. In front of a mirror

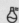

EQUIPMENT
None

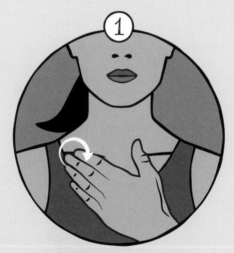

Using flat, closed fingers on the right hand, press firmly into the left collarbone in deep circular motions for ten seconds, working from the center of the chest along the length of the collarbone.

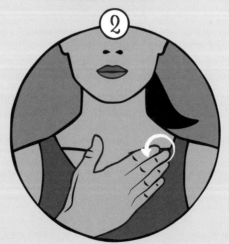

Repeat on the right side of the body.

JAW STROKES

To illuminate skin the emphasis lies in increased circulation to the jawline where toxins can accumulate. Skin quality can be greatly improved with continued stimulation to this area.

Benefits

Sculpts the jawline.
Can improve clarity
of skin.

REPEAT
5 times

TIME
Approximately
1 minute

ENVIRONMENT
Standing or seated.
In front of a mirror

EQUIPMENT
Facial oil or face cream

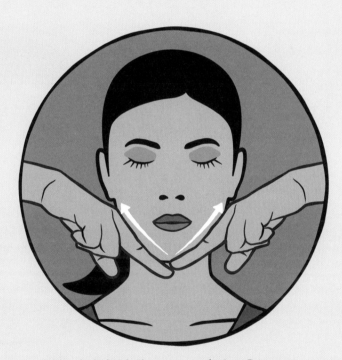

Apply a little facial oil or cream to the jaw. Create two "V" shapes with the index and middle fingers, face down, then place them onto the chin, with the fingers interlaced. Using firm pressure, quickly sweep the fingers up to the ears, keeping the jawline between the index and middle fingers.

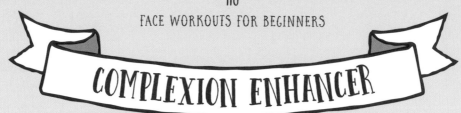

COMPLEXION ENHANCER

Fluid, flowing movements over the face help to tone and illuminate
the skin, which can also become a regular part of a facial routine.

Benefits

Improves tone
of complexion.

REPEAT
5 times

TIME
Up to 1 minute

ENVIRONMENT
Standing or seated.
In front of a mirror

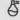

EQUIPMENT
Facial oil or face cream

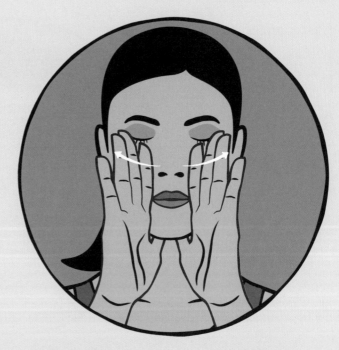

Apply a few drops of facial oil or cream to the face. Align
both index fingers with the nose, with thumbs positioned
under the chin. Using firm pressure, slowly glide the
hands over the cheeks to the outer part of the face.

PINCH AND HOLD: JAW

This exercise concentrates on activating lymph glands to promote oxygenation, in addition to dispersing fluids around the jaw and neck area—imperative for definition to be achieved.

Benefits

Definition to the jawline and increased blood flow.

REPEAT
5 times

TIME
Up to 2 minutes

ENVIRONMENT
Standing or seated. In front of a mirror

EQUIPMENT
None

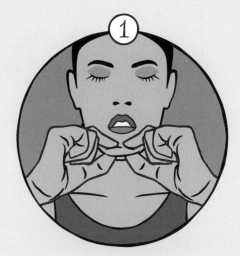

Pinch the chin between the thumbs and index fingers, and hold for five seconds.

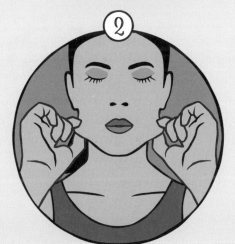

Repeat the action at intervals along the jawline, working toward the ears.

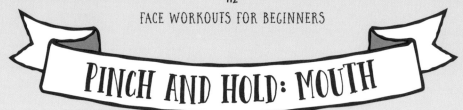

PINCH AND HOLD: MOUTH

Using the pinch-and-hold technique around the mouth helps to reactivate muscles that cause deep lines, including trauma lines.

Benefits
Improves mobility and can soften lines around the mouth.

REPEAT
3 times

TIME
Approximately
30 seconds

ENVIRONMENT
Standing or seated.
In front of a mirror

EQUIPMENT
None

NOTES
The hold time can be increased to 10 seconds on the second and third times if more intensity is required.

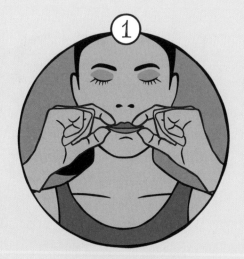

Pinch the outer edge of the mouth firmly between the thumbs and index fingers, and hold for five seconds.

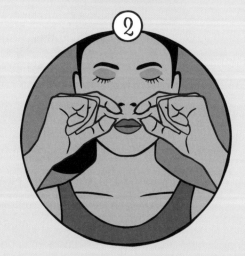

Repeat the pinch along the natural contour toward the nasal passage.

PINCH AND HOLD: CHEEKS

This exercise helps to increase blood flow, leading to more plumpness and illumination to the apples of the cheeks.

Benefits

Improves radiance and fullness in the cheeks.

REPEAT
3 times

TIME
Up to 3 minutes

ENVIRONMENT
Standing or seated.
In front of a mirror

EQUIPMENT
None

NOTES
The hold time can be increased to 10 seconds on the second and third times if more intensity is required.

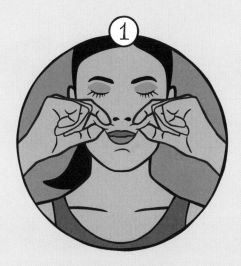

Firmly pinch the area of skin beside the nose where the apples of the cheeks begin, between the index fingers and thumbs. Hold for five seconds.

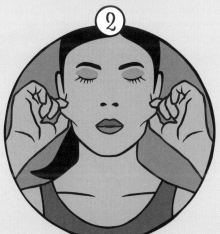

Repeat the action at intervals along the upper part of the cheeks until you reach the ears.

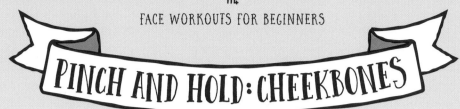

PINCH AND HOLD: CHEEKBONES

Cheekbones are fundamental to the framework of the face.
This exercise intensely manipulates muscles to encourage
mobility and tone over time.

Benefits
Improves definition
and relieves tension.

REPEAT
3 times

TIME
Up to 3 minutes

ENVIRONMENT
Standing or seated.
In front of a mirror

EQUIPMENT
None

NOTES
The hold time
can be increased to
10 seconds on the
second and third times
if more intensity
is required.

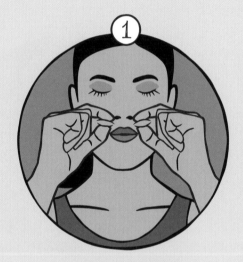

Firmly pinch the
skin under the
cheekbones
between the index
fingers and
thumbs, starting
beside the nose
where the
cheekbones begin.
Hold for five
seconds.

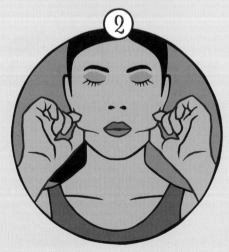

Repeat the action
at intervals under
the cheekbones
until you reach
the ears.

EYE TAPPING

An effective way to move fluid around the eyes and create the sensation of awakening, is by tapping all around this delicate area.

Benefits
De-puffs, improves circulation, and wakes up tired eyes.

REPEAT
10 times

TIME
1 minute

ENVIRONMENT
Standing or seated

EQUIPMENT
None

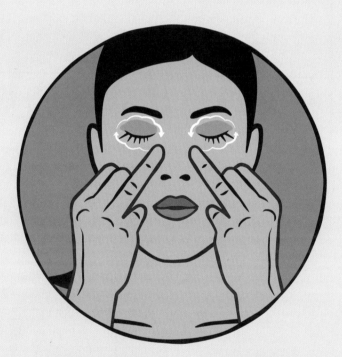

Firmly tap around the eye area with the ring fingers, starting close to the bridge of the nose and moving along to the outer eye, then over the eyelids.

RELAX CHEEKS

Slowly stimulating the cheeks using facial oil or cream is an effective
way to activate blood flow and slow down the mind and body.

Benefits

Relaxes the facial
muscles. Improves
radiance and
plumpness of the skin.

REPEAT
10 times clockwise,
10 times
counterclockwise

TIME
Up to 2 minutes

ENVIRONMENT
Standing or seated

EQUIPMENT
Scented facial oil
or face cream

NOTES
Breathe deeply in this
mindful state.

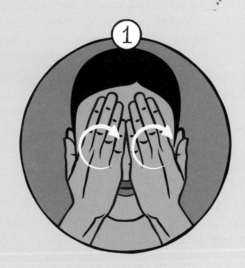

Smooth scented
facial oil or cream
into the hands.
Close the eyes
and cup the hands
over the face to
inhale the scent.
Press the palms
confidently onto
the upper parts
of the cheeks and
slowly move in a
circular motion.
Make ten circles
in a clockwise
direction.

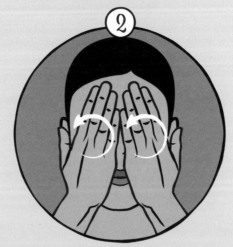

Repeat in a
counterclockwise
direction.

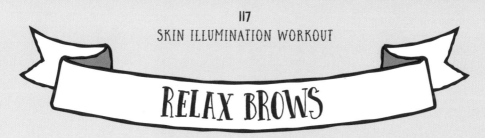

RELAX BROWS

Relaxing the brow area can offer a time to be mindful not to overwork this part of the face, which is vulnerable to creating unwanted lines.

Benefits

Brings awareness of tension or frowning. Can ease tension headaches.

REPEAT
10 times clockwise,
10 times
counterclockwise

TIME
Up to 2 minutes

ENVIRONMENT
Standing or seated

EQUIPMENT
Scented facial oil
or face cream

NOTES
Breathe deeply in this
mindful state.

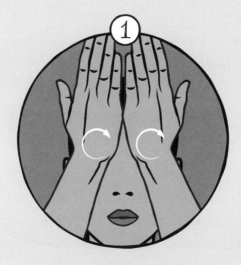

Smooth scented facial oil or cream into the hands. Close the eyes and cup the hands over the face to inhale the scent. Press the heels of the hands confidently onto the brow bones and slowly move in a circular motion. Make ten circles clockwise.

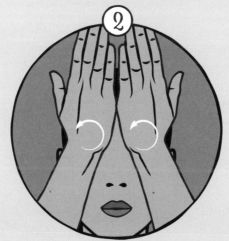

Repeat in a counterclockwise direction.

RELAX FOREHEAD

Relaxing and gently massaging the muscles of the forehead not only assists with easing tension but also brings awareness of how a relaxed forehead should feel.

Benefits

Brings awareness of tensions that cause lines and wrinkles. Can ease tension headaches.

REPEAT
10 times clockwise, 10 times counterclockwise

TIME
Up to 2 minutes

ENVIRONMENT
Standing or seated

EQUIPMENT
Scented facial oil or face cream

NOTES
Breathe deeply in this mindful state.

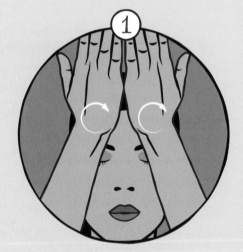

Smooth scented facial oil or cream into the hands. Close the eyes and cup the hands over the face to inhale the scent. Press the heels of the hands confidently onto the forehead and slowly move in a circular motion. Make ten circles in a clockwise direction.

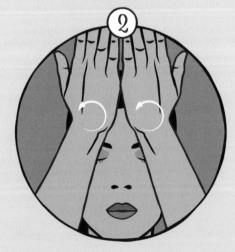

Repeat in a counterclockwise direction.

GENTLE FACE PINCH

Lightly pinching over the face offers gentle stimulation to promote blood flow, which reveals more illumination in the skin.

Benefits

Leaves skin feeling revived, radiant, and plumper.

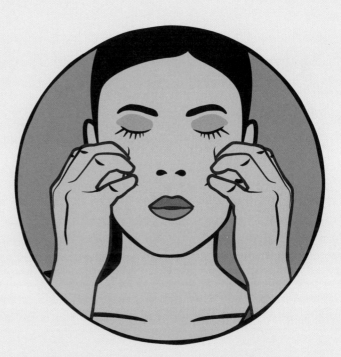

REPEAT

Continuously 3 times

TIME

Up to 1 minute

ENVIRONMENT

Standing or seated. In front of a mirror

EQUIPMENT

Facial oil or face cream

NOTES

Can be performed with eyes closed.

Ensure there is a little facial oil or cream on the fingertips. Using the tips of the fingers, gently pinch over the face starting with the cheeks, over the temples, up to the forehead, over the cheeks, and along the jawline.

NOTES

The exercises have been modified for ease, with no equipment necessary, and can be performed anywhere, so are ideal on a work break or when time is limited.

EXPRESS WORKOUTS

THESE WORKOUTS WERE CREATED TO OFFER A DYNAMIC SEQUENCE OF EXERCISES TO TACKLE TWO COMMON CONCERNS. THE SPEEDY GLOW AND LIFT AND THE SPEEDY DE-STRESS WORKOUTS CONTAIN THE MOST ENERGIZING EXERCISES FOR ON-THE-SPOT RESULTS, AND ARE DESIGNED TO BE PERFORMED AS A WHOLE ROUTINE IN THE ORDER GIVEN.

SPEEDY GLOW AND LIFT

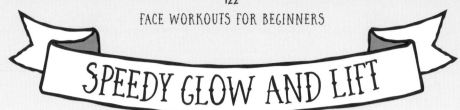

To instantly revive the skin, leaving it radiant and lifted, this workout focuses on increasing circulation in key areas of the face.

Slow Thumb Press

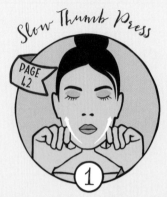

PAGE 42

1

Place the thumbs under the chin and press into the groove between the neck muscles and jawbone, while slowly, continuously, traveling toward the ears. Repeat four times.

Jaw Strokes

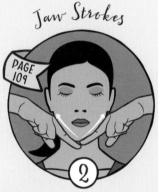

PAGE 109

2

Create two "V" shapes with the index and middle fingers and place them face down onto the chin. Using firm pressure, quickly sweep the fingers up to the ears. Repeat five times.

Pinch and Hold: Cheeks

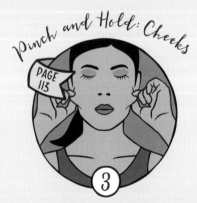

PAGE 113

3

Pinch the skin beside the nose where the cheeks begin. Hold for five seconds. Repeat at intervals along the upper cheeks until you reach the hairline. Repeat twice.

Pinch and Hold: Cheekbones

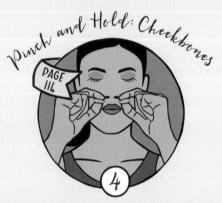

PAGE 114

4

Pinch the skin under the cheekbones beside the nose where the cheekbones begin. Hold for five seconds. Repeat the action at intervals under the cheekbones. Repeat twice.

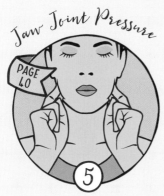

Jaw Joint Pressure

PAGE 40

5

Position the index and middle fingers under the earlobes and press firmly for ten seconds. Repeat twice.

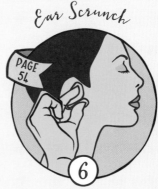

Ear Scrunch

PAGE 54

6

Hold around the edges of the ears with the thumb and fingertips, and scrunch up the ears. Hold for five seconds. Repeat five times, each time scrunching the ear slightly differently.

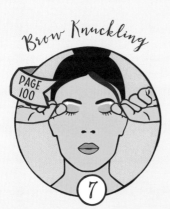

Brow Knuckling

PAGE 100

7

Place the knuckles of the index fingers under the inner brows. Use a firm stroke to pull the knuckles under and along the length of the brows. Repeat twice.

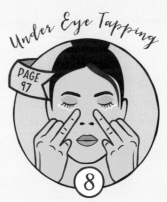

Under Eye Tapping

PAGE 97

8

Using the ring fingers, start close to the bridge of the nose and firmly tap underneath the eye, moving along to the outer eye. Repeat five times.

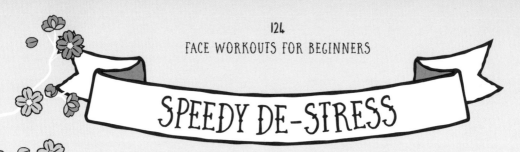

SPEEDY DE-STRESS

This combination of previous exercises encourages a state of calm and relief from tension when time is limited, and can be performed anywhere. Start this workout with Deep Breaths and Shoulder Rolls (see pages 16 and 18–19).

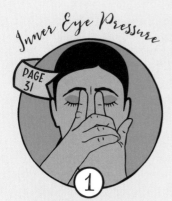

Inner Eye Pressure

PAGE 31

①

Place the index fingers just under each inner brow bone to find the tender spot. Press firmly for ten seconds.

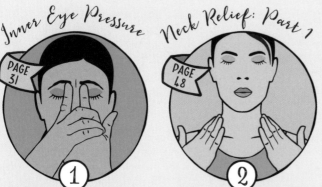

Neck Relief: Part 1

PAGE 48

②

Position closed fingers at the nape of the neck, then press firmly as you move down to the collarbone in one continuous movement. Repeat five times.

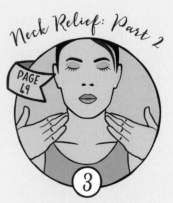

Neck Relief: Part 2

PAGE 49

③

Place closed fingers behind each ear. Press down firmly to the base of the neck. Repeat five times.

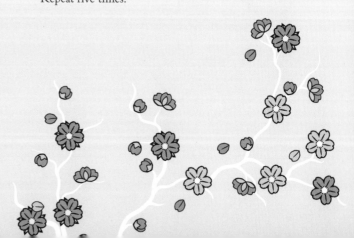

Inflated Cheeks

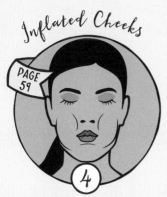

PAGE 59

4

Inflate the cheeks fully with air and hold for ten seconds. Release. Inflate the cheeks fully and hold for twenty seconds. Repeat twice.

Sucked-In Cheeks

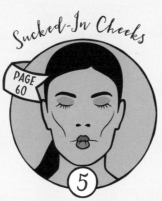

PAGE 60

5

Firmly purse the lips together and suck in both cheeks. Force more suction so that the cheeks are entirely deflated with the lips sucked inward. Hold for fifteen seconds. Repeat twice.

Frown Line Knuckling: Part 1

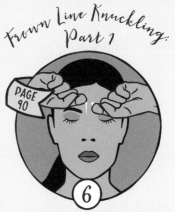

PAGE 90

6

Place the knuckles of the index fingers in between the brows. Press firmly and glide upward in twenty short, quick strokes, alternating between left and right knuckles. Repeat twice.

Frown Line Knuckling: Part 2

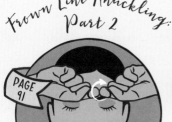

PAGE 91

7

Place the knuckles of the index fingers in between the brows. Pressing firmly, make tiny circular motions. Move the motion from close to the inner part of the right brow, back to the center, then to the inner part of the left brow. Repeat twice.

Temple Massage

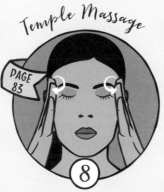

PAGE 83

8

Close the fingers together and place flat fingertips on the temples. Using gentle pressure, apply circular strokes to the temple area. Circle ten times in a forward motion and ten times in a backward motion.

Central Massage

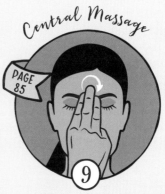

PAGE 85

9

Close together the index, middle, and ring fingers of one hand and place on the center of the forehead. Using firm pressure, move the fingertips in a small circular motion for twenty seconds.

INDEX